Food for Consciousness

Holly Paige

Getting Back on Track of your True Peak Potential

2nd edition
Copyright © Holly Paige 2017
Published by Edenic States.
Cover Photograph by Holly Paige
Cover Design: andrewdaviscreative.com
contact details: info@edenicstates.com

ISBN 978-0-244-04900-3

All rights reserved, No part of this book may be reproduced, in part or in whole, by any means, except for brief quotations embodied in articles and reviews, without the express written consent of the author.

Disclaimer:
This book is sold for information purposes only. The individual retains responsibility for the consequences of acting on any of the information in it. Nothing in this book should be construed as medical advice. Also of course it remains the responsibility of the reader to b sure of the legalities of the use of any food or herb in his or her country of residence.

"This excellent book shows you how to live a happier, healthier, more fulfilled life – in every area."
Brian Tracy – Author – Maximum Achievement

Acknowledgments:
With thanks to my mother Ann Rosemary and my father Geraint Lewis, and to Bruce Barratt, Jasmine Barratt, Bertie Whelan and Elizabeth Paige for their ongoing inspiration.

And to the many people who shared knowledge; also friends who have supported the process in so many ways in all stages. Special acknowledgements to Tony Wright who revealed the biological origins of the fall from grace and made sense of the scientific research regarding the human experience today.

"We are moving into a very different and profoundly preferable state of consciousness"
~ Holly Paige, Food for Consciousness

"Don't ask what the world needs. Ask what makes you come alive, and go do it. Because what the world needs is people who have come alive."
~ Howard Thurman

"To romanticize the world is to make us aware of the magic, mystery and wonder of the world; it is to educate the senses to see the ordinary as extraordinary, the familiar as strange, the mundane as sacred, the finite as infinite."
~ Novalis

In this book you will discover:

how to connect with the life force and bring it into your everyday life
- how you can begin to fulfil your unique potential
- how we as a species can reclaim our true physiology and minds, through rebuilding our neural systems, reading the DNA progressively more accurately and reconnecting to nature and source.
- how to use your mind the way it was intended to be.
- how you can unveil a new sense of self, that feels more like the real you, your true nature and identity connected to the greater life of nature and the cosmos
- the phenomenal new research of the last few decades which changes how science views the brain
- how you can build and fuel your neural system with natural undamaged nutrition that will supply it with the biochemicals it needs for optimal functioning.
- detailed nutrient rich natural food nutrition, that will work in a variety of locations, climates and situations, including minerals, fatty acids and amino acids and what you are likely to be missing.
- specific recommendations to cover the needs of young people and take into account their needs for growth
- tips on making raw food and plant based diets work long term
- give a complete repertoire of delicious, easy, simple and quick raw vegetarian recipes that will supply the vital nutrients

- how to equip your kitchen to be your laboratory of human potential with the biochemistry of ancient forest life.
- highlight effective use of herbs and supplements and powerful techniques to help you expand your state of mind.
- connecting to the earth that is the local source of our physical life and the benefits of doing this
- which bodily cleanses are of most benefit and basics of how to do them.
- how we can change our thinking to engage with the life that is dreamed for us, and is given to us in the form of our destiny
- how to experience that exquisite feeling, every day, of being fuelled by the Life Force itself supported the process in so many ways in all stages.
- point you to the next steps in finding more about this incredible phenomenon.

Contents

Introduction

1. Origins ~ Your Unique Codes for Life
2. What on Earth's going on ~ the Human Story
3. Getting Back on Track of your True Peak Potential
4. Eating the Biological Diet of our Species
5. Brain Biochemicals to Optimise Potential
6. Living in Beauty ~ Natural Lifestyle
7. Cleansing and Regenerating your Body Ecology
8. Reclaiming and Sustaining your Mind
9. Our Hormonal Human Life Cycle
10. Recreating the Psychoactive Forest ~ in your Kitchen
11. Succeeding ~ Bringing the Life Force back into your Life
12. Recipes

References, Reading and Resources
Appendices

Preface Second Edition

Since publishing the first edition I have had plenty of chance to talk to people about the ideas presented in this book. In this preface I want to try to encapsulate these ideas to give a framework and purpose to reading the rest of it.

This book is about how we can live in a different sense of self, one that feels better more suited to life on this planet. It's based on research, both scientific and in the field, in other words in the laboratory of every day life. It looks at the task of every day life almost as an engineering project. I look at the actual mechanics of being human, drawing on science but in a layperson kind of way. It turns out that food, i.e. the chemicals we put in our bodies are a major factor in our discovery of our preferable sense of self, that's why it figures so prominently in the book. To be honest, with a well-adjusted diet, I find myself spending very little time thinking about my next meal. Fine-tuning this part of life leaves us free to enjoy life in a bigger way. The premises of this book is far from a spiritual concept. It's a generic practical proposal for life and regenerating our neural systems to connect us into the mind of nature. Changing our chemistry through food and herbs, adjusting the way we use our minds, reconnecting to natural electromagnetic fields and using some devices and supplements, in a methodical way, it seems highly likely that we can really turn our human trajectory direction we would like to go and become the kind of humans we would like to be.

The basic story is that when we left our natural biological habitat millennia ago we changed our internal chemistry. This happened because of the changed environment and nutrition. The way our bodies and brains are constructed depends not only on our DNA but the way it is read or transcribed and this depends on the chemistry in the body. So now our DNA is not read to its full blueprint. This has affected in particular our neural system, endocrine system, immune system and digestive system. One of the results is that the left and right hemispheres of the cerebral cortex of the brain operate quite differently to each other and somewhat discordantly, giving us a split sense of self. The changes to the endocrine system affect our hormones and the function of the pineal gland. We are dominated by our own sex hormones rather than being bathed in the rich mix of pineal, plant and other human hormones that we once were. Our immune systems are no longer working to full capacity and our digestive systems can no longer break down the food we would have once eaten as part of the natural diet of our species. So even replicating the natural diet requires ingenuity. It's an interesting challenge and an extraordinarily fun one to engage with because it takes us step by step to feeling better in a profound way.

Holly Paige September 2017

Introduction

Food for Consciousness was a surprise for me. When I was looking for that feeling in life that we innately knew we are designed to experience, the last thing I expected to find was a connection with nutrition. Having said that, food is still only one part of the solution. In this book I look at three strands that weave together: nutrition and natural lifestyle, the way we use our minds, and the way we connect to nature and each other. The time has come now in the human story for us to choose whether we live in the ways of the planet thus live our natural lifestyle and survive and thrive, or not. I have looked at the human situation through two angles, one of science and one of mythology. This gives us as a unique sense of perspective. Weaving the two together, and seeing where they match, things come into focus and make sense in a way they never have done before. We see not just extremely revealing data but also a storyline to take us to where we want to go. Some of this storyline can appear to be in the realms of science fiction but the data it is based on are true, the methods have been experimented with and as we know that fiction can come true.

Humans are by nature experimental and this life on Earth is an experiment. The experiment concerning this book is the one of getting back on track of our true peak potential. The approaches proposed are for sure experimental but not as risky as the current experiment taking place on the planet. With the human neural system corrupted, running on a biochemical mix quite different to what it was designed to run on, humans are creating havoc. We see this not just on the news but in our everyday lives and interactions. At the very least we see that people are not living to their full human potential. So the material in this book is proposed as a sane way forward, to regenerate our neural systems as best as we know, to reclaim the use of our minds and reconnect to the bio-electromagnetic field of the planet.

Research in the fields of anthropology, plant biology, mythology, human experience, and on the brain itself, suggests that we could be living in a very different and profoundly preferable state of consciousness.. One that we nowadays glimpse in what we call peak states. The knowledge and ideas presented in this book are chosen to help us shift into an energetic state of mind and body where we can experience true happiness.

The way we eat and our hormonal balance have a huge impact on how we feel, experience life and behave. Through regenerative nutrition, we can all significantly, swiftly and sustainably improve our brain and body chemistry. This enhances our energy, effectiveness, mental acuity, intuition, creative powers, harmonious connection, joy, happiness and sheer pleasure of existence and helps us attain substantially more success in our chosen paths. Ultimately we have the potential as humans to ongoingly experience a sense of well-being now usually associated with peak states 'in a benign state of perpetual wonder and joy', as Tony Wright, author of 'Return to the Brain of Eden' describes it, as 'magical animals' as described by comparative mythologist John Lash.

When you nourish yourself a certain way, the way in fact, the human species is designed to, your mind clears, the neural system rebuilds, neurotransmitter levels flourish and a sense of awareness is activated that simply is not possible without the biochemical foundation in place. Having found this new sense of connection, your perception expands. While food and nutrition remains important , your focus reaches out and, freed from the confines of the analytical mind, to the larger world of nature, to the bigger story of humanity, to live the life of your destiny: adventure, romance, wisdom, beauty and fun. This book is designed to tell you about the food and the nutrition of consciousness, food for consciousness. It is also food for thought, about life and what it can be. It reveals both profound and practical knowledge.

Much of the knowledge here concerns creating a doable infrastructure in your life to begin to recreate the brain biochemistry of ancient memories, in the magnificent forested areas where it seems humans once dwelt. This is not a book about the past, it is very much a book about now and the future, about where we go from here. It is about things to do which we enjoy and love, which make for true joy and happiness. The future is unknown and for us to create with this energy. As we go further along this trail and tune into the intelligent patterning that permeates all life, more answers come.

The key to the door is consistent practical engagement, day by day. As we actually begin to enhance the capabilities of our most crucial resource and tool of investigation, the brain and body complex, we will comprehend things we could not possibly have imagined, and certainly could not have read about in books. By integrating consciousness enhancing nutrients and plants into our bodies and lives in a stable way, we can change our perceptions and the way we do things so that we begin to create a different kind of world. This can happen in a seamless manner that works with the threads of our lives and those around us. In fact increasing harmony is one of the most important aspects of this way of life. Whatever our current situation we can make some kind of positive change which will open doors to more opportunities. Our trust that this will happen helps us to follow our highest energetic feelings.

I cite references for much of the information presented within these pages. Your own experience and research in the context of your own life are what matters. It is for you to try things and see how they work and how they feel. My suggestions are based on what has worked for me and many other people who have worked these methods over the years. Again, it's by consistent application of a combination of the activities, day by day, that you see results. Experiment and find out what works for you, and refine the plan for your individual needs. I continue to be grateful for feedback of what does work and what doesn't.

I became very curious about, 'what is wrong with people' at an early age and spent most of my life looking for the missing pieces. In particular I was puzzled that what people feel, what they think, say and do can be so incongruent. Living in different cultures, the arrival of my children, and the experience of changing to a neuroactive biological diet were pivotal moments in the journey. The search was for that feeling of fulfilment and connection, that we innately know is ours.

For those who are interested I have a degree in physics and a diploma in clinical hypnotherapy but these are just part of a series of subjects that I have studied to put together the knowledge I needed to discover this knowledge about humanity and how to get back on track of being truly human again.

The more expanded our awareness becomes the more mystical and wondrous our experience of the universe becomes. My aim here is to take the mystery out of the information so we can experience more of the real mystery that is life.

Holly Paige
November 2016

1. Origins ~ Your Unique Codes for Life

I begin by describing how we come into this life with unique codes that define us as individuals. One of them is our DNA and reading this code to its full potential blueprint is a major theme in this book.

You come into the world with two unique codes. They make you unique and they hold the keys to your potential. Strangely this is rarely thought about in the times we live in and instead we resort to living by cultural conditioning, the programming that we receive in childhood through those around us. Of course the other people we are influenced by are in the same situation. Cultural conditioning is very limiting and likely goes against everything you innately feel about life, what you want to do and who you are. The reasons this situation came about are deep and we go into them soon.

The real life we came here for unfolds as a mystery because it has become obscured. From the beginning we are encouraged to fir into roles which come out of humanity's conditioned minds. Underneath all this many of us experience yearnings for something more real, that aligns with our deepest feelings.There are many clues. The codes you were born with define your attributes and gifts, physically and mentally and point the way to you living your full potential.

Firstly your DNA is a gift you are born with and remains there through to the end of your life. Even as we grow older, the information to build our physical bodies remains comfortably there. This is a molecular pattern in each cell which holds the information to build your physical body and brain. It connects you to your family and ancestry. In each cell of your body is the same DNA, read differently in different parts of the body and at different stages of life to create the various structures that make you human. It holds the knowledge that organises the microcosm of your physical life. Whatever we are going through it remains there, still holding the knowledge to build you to full specifications. Later in the book I will describe how this code is currently not read to its original blueprint.

The second code places you in time and space, at the moment you were born. Of course this information is generally recorded by calendar dates and clock times. Clocks and calendar measurements originated with something much more solid and absolute, the movements of the Earth through space in relation to the Sun and other celestial bodies. The pattern made by the sun, moon and planetary bodies in the constellations that circle the Earth at the time and place of your birth is another code, a pattern in the sky which defines your connection to the cosmos and to humanity as whole. It places your life story in the grand scheme of things, the macrocosm.

In the times we live, these codes are not belong read accurately and fully and this, I believe is at the root of what we experience today. We are left following programming and conditioning that go against our very natures. What if there are some simple steps you can take, that will begin to change this and immediately make you feel a great deal more fulfilled, more alive, back on track of your true peak potential.

Remember that how the various parts of our bodies and brains are built depends not only on the DNA but the way the information in the DNA is read. This is shaped by the biochemistry in the cell. That's why we can be quite differently built as an adult than as a child. As a species our origins were in tropical forests where all our needs were naturally met. Our food included vast amount of plant material including wild tropical fruit. Human biochemistry consisted not only of our own hormones and other chemical messengers, but also large amounts of biochemicals from the fruits and other forest plants that we were consuming. This is the biochemical environment in which our DNA is designed to be read. Take that away and things change. In the many millennia since we left our natural habitat, the situation has of course complicated itself and there are many steps that need to be put in place. As we begin to put this biochemistry back we can begin to get back on track of reading the DNA blueprint to its full potential.

Nutrigenomics is an emerging science which studies the effects of foods and food constituents on gene expression. I like what Dr Peter Osborne has to say about our DNA in the context of his talks about nutrition and degenerative disease. He points out that the very fact that we are here, after all these generations shows that we all have good genes. He goes on to say that we are having a genetic experience that is reacting to poor choices. I agree with him when he says 'Your genes are a gift'. I would add that they are a divine gift.

Science and mythology tell the same tales in different language. When you bring what the best of them say together it seems that with our neural system operating to full capacity we had once, and can have again, a profoundly expanded sense of perception. Intuition, inspiration, creativity, and a heightened ability to see and make patterns, is our natural endowment. Our desires are meant to healthy, fruitful and rooted in natural imagination. We experienced, and can experience again, cognitive ecstasy.

We are drawn to flickering lights. We see this in the allure of TV and computer screens, tablets and phones. So what were the flickering lights we were drawn to in the forests? The stars above, of course. Not the stars of the movies and TV but the stars in the sky itself. Also the luminescence of nature and the electrical light of the Earth were apparent to us. The songs of the birds, calls of animals, the sound of the wind made sense to us and guided us because we were not stuck in linear logical language. Our imaginations were fired up, and grounded, in nature. From observing the patterns in the stars and in the natural world, mythologies were constructed and we weaved our destinies. It is innate for us to be guided by the stars. Astrology of today, whilst accurate and useful in many regards, has, like everything else, changed. It is read with the analytical reductionist mind that our consciousness today is dominated by, now that we have lost the original reading of our DNA. Just as the medium for fully reading the DNA is a rich mix of human and plant biochemistry, the medium for reading the stars is the state of consciousness that biochemistry produces. An expansive creative, inspired, story telling mode, fluid and inventive, wired into divine imagination. There is more to the story of astrology but that is for later.

As your DNA begins to be read according to its full blueprint you will identify less with your role in the psychodrama of human existence. Your of sense of yourself will change and your natural place in the cosmic order becomes apparent. You stop having to pretend and can be your true self.

2. What on Earth is Going on? ~ the Human Story

In this chapter I zoom out and describe what has happened to humans in terms of leaving our natural biological habitat and the impact this has had on us. From the DNA being read differently, the split in the hemispheres of the brain, and how this has shaped culture, brought ramification after ramification until we have the somewhat dire situation we are in today. The core of the research that underpins this chapter can be found in the book 'Return to the Brain of Eden' by Tony Wright and the writings on the Sophia Myth by comparative mythologist John Lash, which seems to be the most pertinent mythology we have available, much of it based in the Nag Hammadi texts which were discovered in 1945. Science and mythology tell similar stories, in different languages. I also of course draw on human experiences, observations and feelings about what has happened to us as humans and what is still happening now..

So how did this situation that we find ourselves income about? In this chapter I summarise the human story from the point of view of biology, nutrition, brain function and sense of self.

As a young child, life many of us, I noticed that there was 'something wrong with people'. I became convinced it was something to do with the brain, and vowed to find out what it was. As I grew up the question became focused more in my own needs for happiness. I was perturbed by the fact that the things I had thought would make me happy simply didn't. So I began to experiment to find out what genuinely made me feel good. This was really how I got into natural lifestyle. It was noticing how things made me feel. Along the way I got to hear that eating purely fresh raw foods such as fruit, salads, seeds and nuts and so forth made you feel amazing in a way that could only be experienced not described. So of course I had to give it a go. I was stunned. Within 72 hours of eating this way I felt an incredible high. It was like being a child in the garden again! I was intrigued. Why would changing the way we eat make such a huge difference? I was sure again it must be something to do with the brain. A second question came to my mind. How can we increase this feeling, make it even better? And thirdly how could I do this and also be sure that I was fully nourished, in other words how could I sustain this lifestyle? I found the answers I was looking for. They were supplied to me by Tony Wright. In chapter 4 I return to this. For now back to the story. We are in the middle of this story. It began in the legendary Earthly paradise garden, the tropical forests where we were naturally at home. Although it seems there was some kind of paradisiacal experience there has to have been some kind of fallibility at the beginning in order for things to go wrong. Mythological traditions all allude to a time when humans lived in a more exalted state than now, "In a benign state of awe and wonder" after which we fell from grace. Scientific evidence shows that the human brain expanded rapidly until about 200,000 years ago, and then suddenly began shrinking. It seems that these themes are linked. When we left our outer forest environment, we ate differently and our inner environment changed too. The biochemistry of our bodies changed and this affected the way the our DNA is read or transcribed to build us, right from the womb and through our lives. Our brains and bodies began to be formed differently. This meant that our endocrine system began to be formed differently too. The pineal gland began to secrete less of its own hormones. This again affected the way our DNA was read. The differences between the sexes became exaggerated. We lost our connection with the wisdom of nature and replaced it with cultural conditioning. The story goes on. Away from our biological home we eventually developed agriculture. In very recent times we went through the industrial revolution which paved the way for the information revolution and has now laid the foundation for an interesting situation. Although humans have become far removed from their innate lifestyle we now have access to the knowledge of the way back to paradisiacal living. We can move foods around the world and so have access to our natural biological foodstuffs. We have a chance to rebuild our neural system and even create a situation where new generations could be born in a paradisiacal genius state. For individuals who choose it there is a happy story ahead.

The Holy Grail

The Holy Grail, sometimes confused with the Chalice, is traditionally said to be a cup, a dish or a stone with miraculous powers providing happiness, eternal youth or food in infinite abundance. It comes into our story here because of its significance in legend as this sought after object. To me it is significant because it represents the perceptual state we so deeply long to be in, a state of cognitive ecstasy where we can even see the luminous light of the Earth, we have what are now considered paranormal abilities and we experience a sense of connection and knowledge that ensures that everything is alright in a very deep sense. In our current condition we get glimpses of this state, we can experience peak states of one kind or another. The point is we are designed to effortlessly live in these states continually and we still have the genetic potential to do so. And even now it is possible to habitually access what we might call peak states. To me this is the biggest most relevant secret in the world today. We have the latent capacity to live in a very different and profoundly preferable state of consciousness to the one we have considered normal. It's a different sense of self, and one that feels much more right to us.

In the Arthurian legends there are two Grail questions. The first one is what is wrong with humanity. And the second one is how we can serve the Grail. The second question can be interpreted many ways. For me it is connected with finding our true humanity and the sense of self that lives in a sublime state of connection with this Holy Grail. Sometimes we don't know what we don't know and we need to follow our hunches and intuition to find it. The answers we get depend on the question we are asking. When you start asking questions about that you are truly seeking and what you would truly like to experience a whole lot of clues may be presented that you might not have noticed before. And these clues would mean nothing if you did not know what questions you were asking.

The Psychoactive Forest

It seems that human life began in tropical forests. In our warm forest home we had everything we need provided for us: shelter, food, an ideal ambient temperature, electrical connection to the Earth, and all the raw materials we needed to build and fuel our brains or 'lenses of consciousness' to the precise specifications represented in our DNA. The fact that we ate copious amounts of raw fruit (containing seeds) and leaves is significant. The molecules of these foods were undamaged by the heat of cooking and so made pristine building blocks. We had just the fatty acids we needed to construct the nerve membranes and myelin sheaths that insulate the electrical signals passing through them. We had the antioxidants to protect these volatile fatty acids. We had copious amounts of the intact amino acids we needed to build the neurotransmitters. And we had the ideal complex combination of fruit sugars that we needed to steadily fuel our brains.

We also had a subtle and complex balance of natural biochemicals pumping through us that kept us in a sustainable 'switched-on', highly functional, grounded, relaxed and healthy natural high state.

Research by primatologist, Katherine Milton suggests that in the wild we had at least twenty times the micronutrients that we would expect to ingest in civilised life. With all these pieces in place we were able to ongoingly experience what we might call cosmic consciousness; these highly energised states we now see glimpses of during experiences we describe in terms of kundalini, psychedelic or peak states.

So, as humans, we existed at our highest most pristine state so far millennia ago in tropical forests where a powerful cocktail of psychoactive biochemicals from our predominantly fruit diet pumped through our bodies and brains 24 hours a day. These were the psychoactive forests.

What does psychoactive mean? The dictionary definition is 'affecting the mind or mood or other mental processes'. I am using it literally to mean 'activate the psyche'. It is possible to create a way of eating and an environment that do just that. And of course trees are part of this. They provide food, connect to us psychically and provide homes for birds who stimulate our consciousness with their song. So there we have it, the psychoactive forest which includes trees and also that whole infrastructure that we set up in our lives to nourish us and create a happy, healthy state of mind.

As humans we feel at home in places of high vegetation; this nourishes us at every level. We ultimately feel more comfortable and relaxed in a garden or a forest than a tilled field or on a hunt or shopping mall.

Our brain activity is conducted on a physical level through electrical signals via neurons (nerve cells) and chemical neurotransmitters which transport the information from one neuron to the next. There are complex and delicate structures within the neural cells called microtubules which are associated with cognition, intelligence and even higher consciousness. These structures are particularly responsive to a change in the biochemicals around them. For example a minor change in the cellular concentration of melatonin will radically alter their structure.

Flavonoids are the compounds that give fruit their colour. But they are also micronutrients with very special roles to play. Firstly, they are monoamine oxidase inhibitors. What does this mean? Well, the neurotransmitters in our brains are mostly a class of biochemicals called monoamines and they are constructed from amino acids. These include serotonin, melatonin, dopamine and norepinephrine. Monoamine oxidase inhibitors or MAOI's prevent the monoamines being oxidised so keep our monoamine neurotransmitter levels high, in fact in modern times they have been used as anti-depressants. The greater quantities of neurotransmitters in turn stimulated the pineal gland and the production of even more powerful pineal monoamine oxidase inhibitors (MAOI's), such as pinoline which further boosted neuroactivity. A powerful feedback loop involving the pineal gland was thus in operation. In this state the pineal gland pumped out plentiful supplies of melatonin, which enabled us to feel more and have more connection to a more expanded state of consciousness. It also pumped out small but steady amounts of the neurotransmitter, di-methyl tryptamine (DMT), crucial for higher perception. In large amounts this chemical is known for producing overwhelming visions and other impressions. In the subtle amounts we are talking about here, it enhanced our awareness of reality.

Flavonoids also work with our natural steroid hormones including our sex hormones. Hormones are, in short, chemical messengers that operate throughout our bodies and brains. Todays we are to a large extent run by our own sex hormones. In our forest days we were operating on a synergistic combination of our own hormones and the forest biochemistry. The forest was a biochemical factory. The trees that offered the most attractive fruit, that made the early humans feel the most amazing would have been eaten more and their seeds more widely distributed, increasing the prevalence of these trees. This is the symbiotic relationship between humans and fruit trees, a connection we still sense today. We lived in symbiosis with trees. We were literally children of the forest.

The premise that we are designed to live in a mixture of not only our own hormones but forest biochemistry tallies with the mythology about our ancient connections to trees and living within the Earth's bio-electromagnetic aura, also that there is a sacred connection between man, woman and the Earth. Myths tell of the dryads, the tree nymphs, the female nature spirits of the forest. We also hear of the tree of life and the tree of knowledge. The Buddha attained enlightenment under a Bodhi Tree, which was a fig tree. It feels like this is an allusion to this long ago situation. What's more, because the sex hormones were diluted with forest biochemistry, the differences between the genders were less. With testosterone modulated, men had more qualities that would now be more associated with the feminine, in a good way. And oestrogen modulated women had more of the good masculine. Testosterone is not a problem, it is the loss of plant chemistry that would modulate it. We are designed to operate in a mixture of our own and plant hormones, take the plant chemistry away and we are left literally stewing in our own juices.

For whatever reason, possibly a drought that diminished the forests or some other environmental occurrence, or who knows, some idea that got into our heads, we humans began to leave the forests. Although of course there are tribes that today live in tropical forests, they have still been through the process of disruption at some stage. The loss of this heady mix of forest chemistry had a profound effect. It disrupted the pineal feedback loop and even when humans return to the forest it takes more than a change of diet and environment to get it back.

Two Senses of Self

To recapitulate, it is not DNA alone that determines the way our bodies and brains are built. There is another major factor and that is the way that the DNA is read or translated or 'transcribed'. This is epigenetics, how traits are passed down through the way the DNA is read. Nutrients and hormones both have a role to play in this. They determine the accuracy to which DNA is read and the way the body and brain, or 'lens of consciousness', is built, from the moment of conception. This of course affects whether we reach our full genetic potential.

In our original forest home flavonoids from fruit affected the action of our natural steroid hormones including our sex hormones such as oestrogen and testosterone. Without this complex forest biochemistry our sex hormones rule the roost. This affects the way our endocrine system is built and the pineal gland pumps less melatonin and other biochemicals. This has a secondary effect. So there are two major changes in the body biochemistry which affect the way the DNA is read. This affects the way every part of us is built, including the brain. Because of slight fundamental differences between the two hemispheres the left hemisphere build is affected far more than that of the right.

Fast forward to the early years of the twenty-first century and we find researcher Professor Simon Baron-Cohen at Cambridge University, researching autism and showing that high levels of testosterone in the womb when a baby is growing causes retardation in the structural development of the left hemisphere of the neocortex of the brain. He describes his research subject as extreme male brain. This is the point. He is describing an extreme example of something that is already happening. Our sex hormones are running amok. Without the moderating effects of all the fruit chemistry they are causing a structural change to the left hemisphere of the brain.

Most of our impressions of the left and right hemispheres of the brain have been formed by the research of Roger Sperry in the 1960's. Actually in the decades since then some very interesting research has been done which tells us a lot more. But for the moment, back to Roger Sperry. You can read more about his fascinating split brain research online. In short, he found that the left side of the brain currently controls analytical and verbal tasks while the right half takes care of the space perception tasks and music, for example. The right hemisphere is involved when you are making a map or giving directions on how to get to your home from the bus station. The right hemisphere can only produce rudimentary words and phrases, but contributes emotional context to language. Without the help from the right hemisphere, you would be able to read a word but you would not be able to imagine what it is. The right half deals with feeling matters. Hence the great Sperry quote, "The great pleasure and feeling in my right brain is more than my left brain can find the words to tell you."

Since the time of Sperry it has become clear that it's not so much a matter of specialisation. Something has happened to the left hemisphere which has left it able to perform only certain functions - the more logical linear ones, including conceptualisation and language - which are thought of as its specialties. In the last three decades remarkable characteristics have been discovered about the right hemisphere of the brain, which I will outline.

Tony Wright is the scholar who first brought this phenomena to public attention in his book 'Left in the Dark', now republished as 'Return to the Brain of Eden'. In 2007 he even stayed awake for 11 days and nights on what he called a 'primate like diet' (similar to the frugivorous forest diet) to prove his point. I was fortunate enough to witness most of this event and can report that he was coherent throughout. His proposition is backed up with the evidence of recent decades of research in various fields of science. Basically it is that the steroid hormones, in particular testosterone, acting without the modulating effects of the complex plant phytochemistry, plus our own pineal hormones, have had a long term effect on the left hemispheres of the brain to all humans over thousands of years. As Tony says, "This is not a mild condition affecting a few people but a serious condition that affects all of us!" Although the hemispheres were once similar, and potentially could be again, there was always some slight difference between them. For this reason the hormonal situation has had a bigger impact on the left hemisphere than on the right. As a result the left brain has become a less functional version of the right although ironically it has become dominant. This dominance is an accepted fact and is known as cerebral dominance. There is extraordinary latent potential in the right hemisphere waiting to be liberated from this cerebral dominance by the left hemisphere.

Here's some of the key research that adds weight to the proposition. There are more details about this in the Appendices at the back of this book.

In the 1980's Canadian professor Michael Persinger discovered that euphoric or mystical experiences can be accessed when weak but complex magnetic fields are applied to stimulate the right hemisphere of the brain. The same effect cannot be produced with the left hemisphere. An interesting correlation is that certain psychedelic substances do not produce altered states of consciousness in people who have lost the use of the right hemisphere.

In the 1990's Professor Allan Snyder at the Centre of the Mind in Australia began conducting research involving temporarily shutting down the left temporal lobe of the brain using trans-cranial magnetic stimulation. During the experiments enhanced artistic and mathematical ability and improved memory emerged. In Snyder's words: "You could call this a creativity-amplifying machine. It's a way of altering our states of mind without taking drugs like mescaline. You can make people see the raw data of the world as it is. As it is actually represented in the unconscious mind of all of us." A number of Allan Snyder's subjects have reported perceptual changes too – feelings of euphoria and bliss more normally associated with 'peak experiences' and meditation.

The skills that emerged in Allan Snyder's experiments mirror those of autistic savants and also occur in some people whose left hemisphere has been damaged. Darold Treffert, Clinical Professor at University of Wisconsin Medical School, has studied savant syndrome for over forty years. His book 'Extraordinary People' was the first comprehensive summary of autistic savant syndrome and is probably the world authority on autistic savants. In a recent statement he has said: 'I've come more and more to the conclusion that rather than there being right hemisphere compensation, there is rather release from the 'tyranny' of the left hemisphere'

Yet more evidence of the remarkable capacities of the right hemisphere has been revealed by the experiences of neuroanatomist Jill Bolte Taylor. In 1996 she had a severe haemorrhage in the left hemisphere of her brain. Her account tells like a mystical experience. Because mental and physical function is habitually dominated by the left hemisphere, much was initially lost as a result of the trauma of the stroke. However as a result the functions of Jill Bolte Taylor's right hemisphere blossomed.

It seems that when left hemisphere influence is removed mystical sensations and advanced function emerge. So what happens when right hemisphere function is lost?

A fascinating sense of how the left hemisphere of the brain operates when it is deprived of the influence of the right hemisphere is given by the condition of anosognosia. Anosognosia is the name for a condition where a person has a disability and does not know that they have that disability. It occurs as a result of neurological damage and is classically seen in patients who have had a right hemisphere stroke, resulting in a paralysis of the left side of the body. In fact anosognosia occurs in over half of right hemisphere stroke patients (J. Cutting put the figure at 58% in a study described in 1978), while it hardly ever occurs in left hemisphere stroke victims. Some of these patients vehemently deny the paralysis and, in extreme cases may employ defence mechanisms to account for their failure to move the left side of their body. For example if they can't move their left arm they may claim it is just tired or they moved it earlier. Accounts of this are detailed by neuroscientist V. S. Ramachandran. This apparent lying where the person actually believes what they are saying is true is called confabulation. Confabulation can be defined as the formation of false memories, perceptions, or beliefs.

If you are interested, here's a bit more detail about the biochemical process of hormonal retardation of the left hemisphere. Please skip this paragraph if you like, it's not essential for following the rest of the book. It is actually the steroid hormone estradiol that directly retards the structural development of the left hemisphere. Estradiol is made from testosterone by the enzyme aromatase. The process is therefore is affected by the amount of free testosterone available and the degree of aromatase activity. The activity of aromatase is inhibited by plant flavonoids and also the pineal hormone melatonin. As we have seen humans are currently experiencing a deficit of both flavonoids and melatonin. I will come back to the melatonin shortly. For example, the modern human diet provides only about 5% of the micronutrients that other primates ingest each day in the wild. We also probably have about 5% of the amount of melatonin that we would have optimally. (ball park figure) .With an increase in flavonoid and melatonin levels, aromatase activity is reduced and the DNA is read more accurately.

The Pineal Feedback Loop and Other Changes

The initial changes in the way the DNA is read were caused by the change in what we ate and a change in the environment. They affected the way the body and brain are built and the way they run. I have explained the change to the cerebral hemispheres. The resulting limitation to the left hemisphere and its dominance (cerebral dominance) not only affects our perception, it also affects the way the body runs. The changes are many, the most notable are to the neural system, the digestive system, immune system and hormonal/reproductive system.

The digestive system nowadays does not have the power to break down and extract all the fine nutrition from food the way it once did. Our immune system does not currently shake off every bacteria, virus etc that can cause us problems. And our endocrine system in other words our hormonal system is disrupted. This is a whole topic in itself and brings into question the process of puberty, female monthly cycles, menopause and so forth. We go more into this in chapter 9.

The point I want to make here is the effect on the pineal gland which now fails to secrete its own hormones at levels that are ideal. It pumps a small fraction of the melatonin that it was designed to. It also secretes less pinoline, the mono amine oxidase inhibitor (MAOI) that helps keep other neurotransmitter levels up. And its production of DMT (di-methyl tryptamine), an essential neurotransmitter that enables us to perceive patterns both visually and mentally has reduced from a steady small release to occasional release in times of peak experience or extreme stress. The change in the biochemicals released by the pineal gland has itself two kinds of effect. Firstly the biochemical change alters our perception. Secondly it changes the way the DNA is read for a baby in growing in the uterus. This then effects the way the brain and pineal gland are built and operate. And this then affects the biochemistry in the body. So round and round it goes. This is called the pineal feedback loop. It does seem that this loop could be reversed in a methodical way. In chapter 9 I describe the possibility of doing this. The pineal gland has been known since antiquity to be of extra-ordinary significance. If you keep your eyes open you will see pineal gland sculptures in many places. Here is a picture I took in Marazion, Cornwall, also a picture in the Vatican, (reproduced with permission).

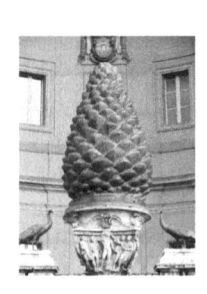

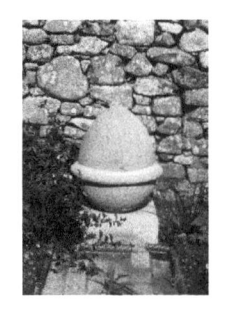

In the appendices you can read in more detail about the relevant brain research of the last few decades.

So what do this all mean in terms of our real life experience? Firstly we have a split sense of self, commonly felt as a split between what we feel and what we think. We also have a split between so-called dreaming and waking lives. Also it's accepted as normal that most of our mental processes are sub-consciousness i.e. we are not fully aware of them. It's a common experience that our state of being can vary from a massive sense of intuitive aliveness to a limited more pondering state. Peak feeling states are inspired, spontaneous, and free flowing where we perceive real time energetic reality i.e. perceiving and feeling how things actually are. Our ponderous states are more rigid, limited, disconnected and fear driven. In such states we are running our lives by ideas or rules. We generally experience life as a mixture of the two. For me it was actually the experience of the change of diet to the one I describe in this book that brought the different states into sharp relief. I was aware that I had shifted to a much more intuitive state and it worked way better for me. It was more functional as well as a more pleasant state to be in. At the same time I was aware of the other troublesome state lurking and ready to take over. This is the split sense of self.

Cerebral dominance exists in all of us, whether in civilisation or in a tribe in the forest, in the city of in the countryside, whether we are right handed or left handed. It does vary slightly in degree from person to person, but compared to how we could ultimately function the differences are splitting hairs.

The left hemisphere has retained language ability. There are language centres in the right hemisphere but as the left hemisphere is dominant the function of language is mainly there. Functions that the left hemisphere has lost are carried by the right hemisphere but, again due to cerebral dominance they are not so easy to access. Feeling is an ability carried by the right brain. Creative, intuitive, artistic, musical and higher advanced mathematical ability are also the province of the right hemisphere because they are beyond the current capability of the left. Because of its limitations the left hemisphere actually needs more rest than the right so right hemisphere function is often accessed through dreams or day dreams. The right hemisphere also has more body awareness and runs the body better. Its restraint by the left hemisphere, as I mentioned, affects our immune systems, digestive systems and reproductive systems, detrimentally. A shift towards the right hemisphere is not just good for our mind state, it is good for our health. It is also looking increasingly likely that, freed from the shackles of cerebral dominance, the right hemisphere could do everything the left hemisphere currently does, including language plus much more besides.

Stimulation of the right hemisphere gives us that sense of the greater reality known as a peak experience or spiritual experience. On the other hand if right hemisphere function is lost, people become increasingly unable to deal with even simple realities of life such as awareness of their own body function or the layout of their own homes. Some teachings describe the two states as the higher self, soul or 'spirit' and the lower self, ego or 'mind'. The left hemisphere or ego has become disconnected from the rest of existence and runs its own story line, which makes us feel separate, potentially in conflict and definitely in competition. It would seem that the left hemisphere has to reduce everything to concepts because it simply does not have the processing power of the right, to perceive things in all their complexities directly.

Looking at the human story over the ages, the left hemisphere concept has been that everything is progressing and getting better. These days, the knowing that something has gone seriously amok is coming to the front of the collective mind and people openly talk about the world having gone mad. The time really has come for this knowledge to come out into the open and be acted upon. The impact of our disconnection is to be seen everywhere, including the general feeling of uneasiness that is the human condition, breakdown in personal relationships, general atrocities, obliviousness to the natural environment and the loss of the once innate sense of the appropriate thing to do in any moment.

There is another component of the problem. The lack of our natural biological nutrition, the nutrients we would get as a matter of course in our biological habitat has a bigger impact on the right hemisphere than the left hemisphere. It has a bigger impact because the right hemisphere retains more complex function which needs this nutrition. Bringing this back in is really the foundation for any improvement. The solution is the subject of the next chapter. Since the problem began millennia ago, not only has the left hemisphere become more limited but it has also become more dominant. Even a few thousand years ago there was more routine right hemisphere access so people had a sense of access to the communications of the divine.

It is not surprising that humans seek out stimulants, relaxants, uppers and chillers, expanders and relaxants. Our brains hunger for biochemicals the way our bodies hunger for foods and our limited left hemispheres create a fearful, needy state. With our neurotransmitters deficient, pineal under-active, melatonin levels lower and left brain structurally limited yet dominant, we see increased aggression, an epidemic in depression and other mental problems, disintegration of social connection and an increase in rules and regulations to compensate for our once innate sense of the right thing to do in any moment. Hormonal imbalances, not surprisingly, are affecting the reproductive system and we also see an increase in many specific health problems due to the breakdown of the immune system and other difficulties associated with a malfunctioning operating system.

The good news is that we can use this information to help us move into a very different and profoundly preferable state of consciousness to the incomplete one that has been considered normal for so long.
There is another part of the story. That's how we get back on track again, how we pick up the story, readjust the biology and experience everything we can hope for and more. In this chapter I looked at how we got here. In the next I look at how we get back on track. The real research that counts is in life itself. Trying things to see how they work out for me and talking with others about their experiences has been a crucial part of the research behind this book. Humans are experimental by nature and life is

inherently a mystery. What I want to do in this book is remove some of the mystery regarding the practicalities of getting into a connected state so that we can be connected into the wonderful mystery of life itself.

So we continue the story of humanity in the context of this biochemical situation. This framework is the one that I use to make sense of life and inspire me as to practical solutions. I have shared the next part, in many classes and talks to give a context regarding the way we eat. I hope it is helpful to you too.

Cooking, Hunting, Plant Medicines, Agriculture, Traditional Diets and Industrial Foods

After we left the forest what would we have eaten? The savanna beyond the forest is mainly grasslands with shrubs. Incredibly adept as we are as a species, we survived and even covered the globe even without our natural diet. Other species removed from the natural habitats don't do so well. For example a panda, removed from the bamboo forests, does not eat well, let alone reproduce. Yet reproduce we did. In fact the loss of the plant phytochemistry and the greater dominance of our sex hormones probably caused human populations to increase though our sense of well being was less. As a species we learned to process the new foods we were encountering that are not really our natural foods. Being incredibly intelligent and adaptable we learnt to process food through cooking and fermenting to remove harmful or indigestible substances in plant matter. As a survival strategy, humans learned to take nourishment by hunting animals and, later, piggy backing off grazing animals by using their milk. These grazing creatures *were* in their biological habitat. They thrived on the grasses, herbs and insects, so their milk was a good emergency measure.

As all this unfolded and we lost our fruit and pineal hormone high, the stronger psychoactive plants became important for reconnecting us to natural wisdom, cognitive ecstasy, and that expanded ecstatic sense of self. Research shows that only the right hemisphere responds to psychoactive plants. Graham Hancock, Terence Mc Kenna and others have suggested that we developed our intelligence through our experiments with the plant medicines. I am looking at things in a different way here, based on the model of the biological origins of the fall from grace, explained in 'Return to the Brain of Eden'. The psychoactive medicine plants were just reconnecting us to what we had already had through our relationships with the fruit trees. As our neural system declined we needed stronger biochemicals to reactivate it. We can experiment with this and experience some residual effects even today. By cleansing and eating a very pure fruit and plant based raw diet we can experience a high with less need for stronger stimulation.

There was a parallel situation going in with our nutrition. As our digestive systems began to be constructed less optimally our ability to extract the nutrition from food declined. So not only had we lost our biological diet but out ability to absorb nutrition in general decreased. Other foods became necessary. In the forest insect material was an automatically part of our diets because it was actually in many fruits in the wilds as well on other vegetation. This was an intrinsic part of our nutrition. Take it away and we need to replace it with something else. Animal and fish flesh would cover these components. Eating them though did increase the steroid hormone and accelerated the decline of our neural function. We had moved into survival mode and did whatever we could to get by. Although the milk of other mammals is not part of our original biological diet we do have the mechanisms in place as we always drank our mother's milk as children. Drinking other animals milk was a way of getting the nutrition from the grasses, herbs and insects that they ate and the sunlight they absorbed grazing naked where we did not. Fermenting them made them digestible even for adults who are not designed to drink mammal milk. Agriculture began around twelve thousand years ago. Humans began to cultivate grains as well as other foods and so needed to live settled rather than nomadic lives. It really is quite incredible the way we as a species developed cultural cuisines that attempted to cover the nutrition that was originally provided for free in our forest homes.

When Dr Weston Price, the famous dentist travelled the world in the nineteen thirties visiting many of the last groups of people whom the roads had not reached. He found people who were happy and optimistic, physically well formed and free of degenerative disease. He catalogued what he found in his book 'Nutrition and Physical Degeneration'. Of course life was not perfect, if it was we would not have degenerated into the state of things now and of course there were many problems in the world in the nineteen thirties. The point is that these people in these studies were so well formed. Weston price found that natural beauty was shared by all the people, putting to rest the idea that beauty is something elitist. He also noticed that people living in the same tribes often looked like brothers and sisters, suggesting that the differences between us may be exaggerated from epigenetic and nutritional factors. He found people with little or no tooth decay and well formed jaws and cheekbones, with plenty of room for the teeth to grow straight and uncrowded. The state of the teeth corresponded with similarly good overall bone structure and also lack of degenerative disease.

The Weston Price studies are exceptionally valuable in what they reveal about human nutritional needs. The groups he visited it were geographically separate and living in quite different situations. It seemed on first glance that what people ate varied enormously from place to place, based on what was locally available , but on close study it became clear that there were some distinct commonalities.

So what are these commonalities? All the people studied ate a large percentage of their food raw, in other words, undamaged by heat. This included raw animal fats. Nearer the equator, in the tropical regions, this would be mainly plant foods, for example tropical fruits, including coconut with it's beneficial fatty acids. At the other end of the spectrum in the far northern latitudes, the Inuit relied heavily on animal fats. This way of eating and living is no doubt more challenging than living in warmer climes, and the life expectancies weren't as long. And yet these people continued through generation after generation with health that would be enviable to many today. Of course there were no refined or denatured foods such as refined sugar or flour; canned foods; pasteurised, homogenised, or low-fat milk; artificial vitamins or artificial additives and colourings in any of these diets. They also ate seasonally and locally. In traditional diets, seeds, grains and nuts are soaked, sprouted, fermented or naturally leavened in order to neutralise naturally occurring anti-nutrients in these foods, such as phytic acid, enzyme inhibitors, tannins and complex carbohydrates. Total fat content of traditional diets varies from 30% to 80% but only about 4% of calories come from polyunsaturated oils naturally occurring in grains, pulses, nuts, fish, animal fats and vegetables. Traditional diets contain nearly equal amounts of omega-6 and omega-3 essential fatty acids. The rest of the fat is in the form of saturated fats such as coconut and animal fats and monounsaturated fatty acids such as those in olive oil. Dr Weston Price reportedly said that he would have loved to find traditional cultures where people lived from only plant foods, but he did not. Now that we have access to supplements and other foods that were not traditionally available it is more viable to avoid animal foods, which is helpful to the growing number of vegans. In the days before globalisation people ate all kinds of things that would seem strange now. It's important to bear in mind, that even though the Weston Price diets are very healthy by today's standards they were still only survival diets, not the optimal human diet. In tribes that consumed more animal flesh and blood and less fruit and vegetables there was a noticeable tendency for more aggressive tendencies.

Primitive diets studied by Dr Price contained at least four times as much minerals and ten times the fat soluble vitamins from animal fats vitamin A, vitamin D and vitamin K2 as the average modern diet. We could compare this to the statistic from the studies of Katherine Milton that a primate in the wild today consumes more than fifty times the micronutrients as the average human in civilisation.The actual numbers of people malnourished on the planet are far higher than the official figures. Most of humanity is malnourished and feeling it. Even obesity is a symptom of malnourishment as overeating is so often an attempt to get the missing nutrition. This is the true picture of world hunger, and one that can be alleviated with intelligent strategies, regarding what we grow and the way we grow it.

A particularly heart warming aspect of these traditional diets is that most make provisions for the health of future generations by providing special nutrient-rich foods for parents-to-be, pregnant women and growing children. Fat soluble vitamins plus many other nutrients are particularity crucial for growing bodies who have not the built up the resources of an adult body. Proper spacing of children and teaching the principles of healthy diet to the young also helped.

It really is so fortuitous that Dr Weston Price documented these peoples at that time. The pictures in his book 'Nutrition and Physical Degeneration' include comparisons between people in the same family. Some were still eating traditional diets and some had moved onto the modern diets brought in by the new transport systems of the time. It is startling noticeable how those eating the new industrial foods had crooked teeth, less well formed faces and looked less happy. Industrial foods dealt a big blow to health. Since then of course we have come a long way. A descent into junk food for many.

We are now seeing a resurgence in interest in healthy eating. We now can move foods around the globe. Whatever we think about air-miles, the reality is that now we have the opportunity to access more of our biological foodstuffs even though we may be a long way from our natural biological habitat. Also we have supplements and superfoods available to us, which while they could be seen as a strange space age way to eat, can be part of the bridge to us recovering ourselves. In time we can ground this way of eating so that we produce foods more suitable for our human needs in our geographical locations. Citing just one example there are varieties of fig tree that will grow in temperate climates.

I want to add here a point that is often overlooked and crucial to make at this point. Although the characters in the Weston price studies who had not begun to eat processed foods were in better shape than the average person in modern culture this did not mean that there were living the highest possible existence available to humanity. It could be said that they were doing an excellent job with survival diets, far form our original biological home. The human spirit is an amazing thing. These Weston Price diets still miss the vast amount of neuroactive compounds once available to us. To create new ways of eating, taking into account the commonality of the Weston price diets and what we now know about the human neural system and our origins is what excites me. Who knows, it may be that even in the tropical forests we ran out of fuel for our expanding brains. e are now in a new phase of discovery as a species.

In Chapter 4 I get into the practicalities of recreating a natural biological way of eating. Now I'm going to look at what has happened to us mentally, which of course is tied up with what has happened to us physically, nutritionally and hormonally.

What does Cerebral Dominance mean for us?

As I have described, the anomalous situation of our split brains mean that we have two sets of perceptions running along side each other; two senses of self, intertwined. It also explains why our thoughts are so often disconnected from our feelings. The mental activities of the left cerebral hemisphere or 'left brain' have become disconnected in many ways, from our feelings, from our surroundings and from higher sources of wisdom. They have gone off on their own stories, unchecked. Left brains are easily programmable; they go round the same programs, beliefs and thoughts again and again, until some intervention happens. These programs are often alien to us, to what we are as humans, what truly works for us and what we want in life. They can be completely senseless, with no purpose and no real value. Much of the work done in therapy is to free people of these programs. In Gnostic mythology this phenomenon is described in terms of mind parasites called the archons. This term was brought into modern public awareness by comparative mythologist John Lash.

Meanwhile, hidden away, there is still right hemisphere function. Originally left hemisphere function was similar to right brain function, the two hemispheres worked harmoniously together and we had whole brain function, rather than split brain function.

'Right brain skills…represent latent but dormant skills that are released from the "tyranny of the left hemisphere," or, more simply, left cerebral dominance in most persons.'
Darold Treffert MD

The right hemisphere is restrained not only by the dominance of the left hemisphere but also the malnourishment that has become the norm for humanity. This nutritional lack has a bigger impact on the right hemisphere than the left hemisphere because its specifications are greater, as it remains a more complex piece of machinery. When people start to nourish themselves with the copious amounts of fatty acids, amino acids and fruit compounds that the right hemisphere is craving, they tend to experience noticeable shifts in perception as if long forgotten parts of them are coming to life. In Chapter 5 we go on to look at techniques and lifestyle practices to awaken this dormant right hemisphere. For now, on with the story.

The Gender Rift

A twist in this story is the separation in the sexes, how male and female became so at odds with each other and so different. The rift is described in mythology and it can also be described biochemically.

The problem is that testosterone in humans is now insufficiently unmodulated by plant and pineal biochemicals. Because of this it is converted by the enzyme aromatase into estradiol. This is called aromatisation. Estradiol plays an important part in the damage to the left hemisphere. Because there is more testosterone in males than females there is more damage to their left hemispheres. If we were still immersed in forest plant and pineal biochemistry then this aromatisation process would not be taking place so it would not be a problematic issue that men have more testosterone. We are talking about an anomalous situation. Men have been affected more, through no fault of their own. Their left hemispheres are more affected than women's and they are more left brain dominant. On the other hand, men have less connections between the hemispheres through the corpus callosum so have extra opportunities to experience a pure right brain state of consciousness. Of course there are new environmental complications arising through female hormones in the environment feminising men, and also further altering women's hormonal state. Basically the glitch in the way the DNA is read has affected the genders differently and has exaggerated the differences. The continued lack of plant and pineal hormones and the predominance of sex hormones means that the genders live day to day in an exaggeratedly different chemical environment from each other. This is something that can be changed radically even in our lifetimes now, with the change of lifestyle practices described in this book. Ultimately women, as the ones that grow babies, have the power to put this situation right, if we can find away to recreate the optimal biochemical environment for a baby growing in the uterus.

Disconnection from the Life Force

The loss of plant and pineal biochemistry and the loss of feeling in the left hemisphere weakened our erotic connection with nature, the Earth and each other. I use erotic here to mean pleasurable feeling which can include, but is not limited to, sexual feelings. Nowadays, because what has happened humanity in general is most likely to experience heightened erotic feelings in the context of sexuality. As humans moved around the world the building of shelters was necessary in many places they found themselves. Possibly climatic changes have played a role too. Not realising what we were missing, we cocooned ourselves from the forces of nature and losing connection with the wisdom of the Earth we replaced it with cultural conditioning. As time went on we developed floors which insulated us against the electrical current of the Earth. Shoes with insulated soles cut us off from Earth connection even outside. As humans cleared forests to grow the new foodstuffs that we had become accustomed to, we eliminated species that did not obviously serve us, We became the dominant force. Eventually we even replaced the natural lights of the sky with artificial electrical lights. In the West in particular, we have become 'safe' from fierce creatures and wild weather. However, we don't feel truly safe or inspired. We took ourselves outside the setting of the grand and majestic natural world. Instead of looking out of ourselves to the Earth, the trees, the animals and the sky, we became self-absorbed; more interested in our own minds than the mind of nature. It was really the forces of fear and control that had us doing this but the results are a greater sense of insecurity and an unnamed loneliness, with the loss of the feeling of being held in the life force. Narcissism, over concern with the self, and co-dependence, or over concern with others, took hold. Both really come from a lack of true sense of self, two sides of the same coin.

Neurotic, in other words ill-adjusted to our environment, having lost our sense of connection to the life force and the wisdom of nature, modern humans can easily feel like victims of circumstances. Having lost many of our innate abilities, and not even knowing what we are capable of has added to this sense. It is true that we are in circumstances now that came about due to forces bigger than us. The problem with victimage is when suffering is raised to be a virtue rather than looked on as something to be avoided. One of the problems that perpetuates this is that a sense suffering actually has social currency. In the words of John Lash "Victimage works because it makes the force of suffering look stronger than the life force itself."

The remedy is connection with the life force, in every way possible. The most important thing to find is our place in the natural world and our wonder of it. This is what gives us a sense of our lives and our place in life. The disconnection is the biggest problem we have.

From Dreaming to Animism to Redemption

In our whole brain state we felt our connection to source and lived in a highly functional state of waking dreaming, in harmony with our natural surroundings. We were part of nature as much as the other species, albeit with extraordinary abilities. As this affliction to the neural system took hold we became disconnected from our natural environment, and wisdom began to be perceived as something separate to us. Spirituality began to be felt as existing 'somewhere else'. This induced a fear state, a fear generated by no longer having the confidence of being connected to the source of our lives through nature. With fear comes a need to control, to keep things familiar so we can understand what is going on. We began to live by superstition rather than the supernatural And by rules, and by the programs running in the left sides of our brains.

Animism could be described as the first kind of emerging religion of humanity. All the natural world is alive and sacred, with 'the belief in a supernatural power that organises and animates the material universe'.

This was and can be a very real experience. As time went on and the actual energetic experience became weaker, spirituality and religion became more mental, more conceptual. At first religions continued to have a nature base but as time went on they became more manmade. Humans projected their need to control onto the source of life and created in their minds an authoritarian, often anthropomorphic God who wanted to control us. The left hemisphere is not creative in the way the right hemisphere or whole brain is. It's creations are based on mimicry or repetition. Right hemisphere or whole brain creativity has a more dream like quality, similar to the fractal self-similar emanations that occur naturally through the life force. From the view of the limited left hemisphere, humans imagine a god with these mimicking qualities, creating in his own image. In this way of thinking, God creates humans in His own image. Then following this logic, these humans create in their own image. We have the idea of creating in the image of god, and the idea of the perfect human that we emulate. In the living world there is actually massive variety within the fractal forms of nature and this applies to humans too. Our programmed beliefs about perfection and being in the image of God are at odds with what we actually experience in the natural world and in our own natures.

As we lost feeling due to loss of neural function we lost our direct sense of connection with the wisdom of nature and the life force As the left hemisphere became increasingly retarded and dominant our minds became dominated by concepts rather than a sense of real time energetic reality. Humans created a god in the image of the left hemisphere, a god that likewise creates in his own image, a kind of replication. So called redemptive religion began to replace the nature based animistic beliefs of our ancestors. From this 'power over' mentality new beliefs emerged such as 'we create our own reality'. Going along with the idea that we are created in the image of an all powerful god who creates everything that somehow we create everything too. The truth is nearer to we co-create together with the source of our reality. Ancient myths describe an originator and a situation of divine emanation, where we are continually dreamed into existence, similar but not identical forms are brought into existence through this process. The emanations have a divine quality of fractality, based in the Golden Mean and Fibonacci series.

In our cerebrally dominated minds, the story goes that as we cannot keep God's rules (in other words our authentic right hemisphere awareness cannot conform to left hemisphere conceptualisation) a messiah is sent to save us, with cost to himself of great suffering. Of course this doesn't work out and we head for a great day of judgement. Belief in a day of judgement, a doomsday, an apocalypse, when judgement is pronounced because humanity still can't get it right has been etched into the human psyche, even amongst folk who say they are not religious. Of course we do need to learn to live in alignment with the ways of nature but this is not for fear of being judged as bad but because unless we do so it may become mechanically impossible for us to thrive on the planet.

The romanticisation of suffering is very much part of our culture. It is even a social currency; we are subtly rewarded for it. People compete to be seen as the victim so they will be thought of in a favourable light. This has been documented in many self-help writings. It's very detrimental to our wellbeing and our ability even to help others, because everyone is competing to be seen as the victim. That is not to deny that people can be victims of things that happen. The point is that the priority is to empower ourselves and those around us as far as possible so this happens as little as possible. In the words of comparative mythologist John Lash "The divine victim mirrors to humanity, not the solution to our suffering and a way to overcome it, but our total, consuming enslavement to it." The best way to help ourselves and to help each other is to live our lives to the fullest potential we are able. This naturally includes helping each other, not to our detriment but in a way that feels good.

The situation became more complicated as time went on and the story unfolded.

In the early days of humanity, with our innate sense of the appropriate thing to do at any moment, we could operate as sovereign beings. Our needs were met by nature and we easily and harmoniously connected with each other for the sheer pleasure of it. Robert Lawlor describes the behaviour of the aboriginal population of Australia in his book "Voices of the first Day". He speaks of humans as walking mystics. He even describes how the spiral motion caused by walking affects our brain states. In time, tribes banded together to help each other and protect themselves. At first they retained a strong connection to the land but human tribal structure developed into mental domination and patriarchy. It became hierarchical and divisive, and warlike. This momentum gathered with the conquests around two thousand years ago in Europe and the Americans five hundred years ago. All of our ancestors were once indigenous people who have been conquered. In time we moved into the kind of political situation that we experience today. You could look at it as a kind of lunatic asylum. As Tony Wright says, this is not a mild condition suffered by a few, but a serious condition that we all have. Moralising achieves little; we need a remedy for the madness. The horrors we hear about in the news such as war, horrific pollution and abuse are the product of the disconnection. Lack of empathy means that individuals do not feel for the pain they cause others. The fear and need to control, and the divisiveness of mental concepts lead to conflict and war. The sense of separation from the Earth, nature and Source leave the more damaged humans with little concern for the Earth that provides for their physical needs and their sanity. As individuals we witness this on a personal level in every day life.

About Dominator Culture

We are designed to operate in a mixture of our own and plant hormones, take the plant chemistry away and we are left literally stewing in our own juices. When we lost that biochemistry there was massive hormonal disruption. Here I want to show how the aberrant chemistry creates a situation where the masculine seems to be a dominant force, and we get the situation known as patriarchy.

The problem we have is that the testosterone in men and oestrogen in women is insufficiently modulated by plant and pineal chemicals. Adding abundant plant foods and melatonin helps, but is not enough to remodel the basic structure of our neural system once it is formed. The unmodulated activity of testosterone has created the left hemisphere of the brain the way it is today. This change affects both men and women, but it affects them differently. In addition to the structural change, there is an ongoing chemical imbalance until we reinstate a truly natural diet suited to our species, and get the pineal gland operating to full potential again. The chemical change plus the structural changes caused by the chemical changes together underpin the dominator culture. Testosterone increases aggression and the need to compete. This affects everyone but men more so. Unmodulated oestrogen in women, especially younger women, tends to make them more compliant. As men have more testosterone than women then a feature of this dominator culture is that men tend to be more dominant and women more submissive. Moral judgements about the situation do little to change it and are really part of the same syndrome. What can change it is a biochemical and lifestyle improvement. Tony Wright calls it 'molecular engineering'.
The patriarchal God, the powerful, controlling, judgmental, paternalistic figure of redemptive religion is of course an aspect of dominator culture. Dominator culture is one of the results of the glitch in the way our DNA is reading it affects us all. This glitch affects our entire neural system, endocrine system, digestive system and immune system and so of course it affects our mood. It is behind the excess levels of fear and anxiety, our doubts, depressions, feelings of disconnection and so on. The further we have moved as a culture from our natural way of life the more extreme this phenomenon has become, whole cultures have been built on it and spread, setting into motion an emotional plague, as Wilhelm Reich called it. It is contagious and has been carried by conquering tribes and nations

who have taken over land previously occupied by humans who lived until comparatively recently in relative harmony with the land. The very fact the self-help movement exists is testament to the state of things. Even the traditional spiritual practices were designed to treat the condition we are born with. If there was no glitch we would be content just to be and with experiencing the wonders of being alive.

Commercialisation is one of the latter day symptoms. It's interesting that it was Edward Bernays, a nephew of Freud who was a driving force behind the advertising industry of the twentieth century. Human feelings were portrayed as dangerous and to be overcome. Our desires were to be directed into the buying of goods that we were persuaded would meet those desires. Money exchange has become entrenched into every aspect our lives, it's just one of the characteristics of the age we live in, part of cerebral dominance is that it becomes like a game.

Correction and Intervention

The industrial revolution made way for the information revolution and whatever problems this has caused there's no doubt that developments in transport and communications have 'made the oceans shrink'. There has been an opportunity for extensive and rapid information exchange, access to scientific research and communication between individuals. In the thick of it I think it has been difficult to fully appreciate what has been going on. In fact there is now so much information that the job is to pick out what is relevant to where we want to go. We now know much of what we need to know to begin restoring human consciousness. As we progress and our awareness increases as result, we will know more. The time has come to focus on solutions beyond the problems. The peoples of the world need to put their heads together. For example, the indigenous peoples of places such as South America are so much more intact in their lifestyles and attitudes in general than the majority of Europeans who have been relentlessly conquered over a long time span. The indigenous healers have so much to help us with so much to teach the industrialised countries. On the other hand it may fall to some of the people who have been industrialised longest to make a stand about the direction we go as humans now, because they have seen where the road goes, they have seen the tricks and some of them are no longer so easily seduced by the modern hype. It's natural for humans to be trusting, we were not designed to deal with this situation. We are now at a time where we must exercise great discrimination in the way we trust and also fulfil our desires.

We are out of our natural habitat and disconnected from natural wisdom. Coopted is a word that can be used to describe it. Co-optation means taking something from its original setting and adapting or distorting it to ends it was not meant to serve.

We are now at a pivotal point. It has become obvious that if we are to thrive or even survive on this planet we need to adopt the ways of the planet. Gnostic myths told of this time, diorthosis, parting of the ways. There is a split within ourselves. We each as individuals need to choose between living the ways of the planet and rediscovering our true humanity or following some other path. It's almost a battle to be human. Without a sense of connection to Source, and unable to trust any artificial authority to do the right thing, people can be quite overwhelmed thinking they have to orchestrate everything themselves. This is not our job. We need to be part of the whole solution but we only need to play our part in it. There are larger benevolent forces than us to orchestrate things. We actually cannot function at our best without connection to divine intelligence living through us. We can find our sense of dominion in our own unique contribution. There are many things we can do to help us find this sense of connection to the benign forces greater than ourselves and to the life force itself. The practical ideas in this book are primarily aimed towards this. The side effects in terms of increased health and happiness come as part of that package.

The point of view of Tony Wright is that although the hormonal damage has been mainly to the left hemisphere of the brain, the right hemisphere has been slightly affected too and its degeneration continues through the generations. We have a window of time at this point in the human story to act, before the right hemisphere too, degenerates to a point where we become dysfunctional beyond repair. Hence the sense that these are end times with a sense of do or die.

Mythology has something to say on the subject too. Hindu mythology tells of four ages over many thousands of years. The cosmic ages run in sequence, from past to future, like this: the best times, all around (Satya Yuga),the better times, mostly excellent (Treta Yuga) the good times, but going bad (Dvapara Yuga) the declining times, going from bad to worse (Kali Yuga). Beginning with the Golden Age or Satya Yuga when we lived in a paradisiacal sense of connection and moving through the Treta Yuga and Dvapara Yuga to the Age of Kali, an age of degeneration and delight, where we are now. It can be hard going but we also have the greatest possibility for individual spiritual progress, partly because we have to work so much out for ourselves. Life spans are comparatively short in this age and we begin to degenerate shortly after puberty (which comes early as I will explain later) before we are even fully developed. Our neural systems continue to develop until at least our fifties and probably longer. So we are degenerating before we are even fully developed. We need to make effort if we want to stay youthful. Time is at a premium for us now and ever more so.

In the Age of Kali we need to work hard for the things we want. In many ways it's a time of closure, even regarding our identity. We are tying up the loose ends of the past to make way for a new way of living, a new way of being. We cannot unravel what has been done over the ages, but we can become a new kind of human. We may have surprises in the way that the Earth can heal what has been done. An encouraging example is the way that fungi will eat up radioactive elements after nuclear accidents. We simply do not have the powers to do these kinds of things that only the Earth can do. The solution for us is simpler than the problem. We can focus on sorting ourselves out and making the connection to divine intelligence. In terms of our potential it's as if we are looking so far back through the circle into the past that we are looking at the future ! What we see as distant past has actually come full circle into our future.

In these times it is very difficult to tell what is genuine and authentic. We are disconnected from our true feelings and our minds confuse us. In fact, the knowledge of our brain state, the anosognosia and confabulation described as a result of cerebral dominance, confirms this. The Gnostics of antiquity described the situation as error beyond the scale of self-correction. We are designed as humans to experiment, and we love to do so, you only have to watch children at play to know this. We are designed with a capability to do things beyond instinctive programming and we can make errors. We are also endowed with a self-correction mechanism and that is feeling, our intuition. The problem is that we find ourselves with limited access to our feelings and intuition.

Although there are methods to regain our innate senses we are actually in need of intervention to get us back on track. What's more we are required to participate in this intervention. How do we recognise genuine benign intervention? Good question. There has been at least one problematic intervention in human affairs in human mythology. Benevolent intervention does not try to make us something we are not. It helps us become who we truly are. It does not ask us to sacrifice or suffer unnecessarily but helps us to shine.

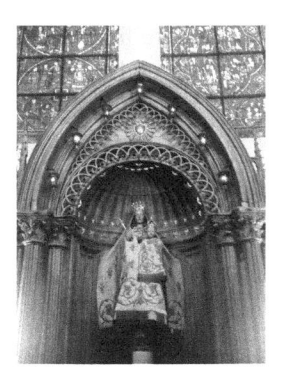

51

There was a vulnerability from the beginning in humans, otherwise things could never have gone so wrong. It could be that we can now come back much stronger as a species. For one thing we are learning discernment. On the biological level it could be that we could get our neural structure to a point where it would not be possible for it to fall apart in the same way. This is speculation right now but an encouraging thought.

How do we know when we are getting back on track? It feels genuinely good, we feel better, we feel more alive. We feel more warmly towards others, we feel more connected to nature. We feel our energy and enthusiasm rise. Benevolent intervention is helpful and kind. It comes from the divine intelligence. It comes in a friendly manner, rather than standing over us or commanding us from a position of authority.

In the next chapter I present what I have found out about three strands of correction in terms of physical, mental, and energetic connection. This is work in progress. As we put what we know into operation, more reveals itself. You could look at some of the proposed courses of action as in the realm of science fiction, the data are real though and as we know fiction can come into reality, and is in fact doing so already. In this case the story is about a very happy future for humans, for those who select it. It is highly likely that in days of old, when the brain was less damaged seers had a more of a sense of things than is possible today and they saw how it would inevitably unfold. The Age of Kali is said to end in 2216, when the sun at winter solstice aligns with the centre of the galaxy. This is an astronomical rather than speculative event. That would tally with around seven generations of hormonal adjustment. Just a thought.

References and Further Reading for this Chapter

Two sources stand out amongst many when researching the human situation. Both scholars, one focused on science, the other in mythology, although both knowledgeable in both subjects.

Tony Wright, author of "Return to the Brain of Eden", is an independent scientific researcher who describes, what he calls the biological origins of the fall from grace. He catalogues how our removal from our ancient original forest home led to a cascade of events including the loss of pineal gland function, a disparity between the left and right hemispheres and corresponding impact on the digestive system, hormonal system and relationship between the genders, immune system and of course function of the brain and our intelligence as well. The corresponding state of mind is depicted here in this painting Expulsion from the Garden of Eden by Masaccio. Through eating our biological diet, 'molecular engineering' in Tony Wright terms, clever adjustment of our biochemistry including judicial use of plant medicines' and a focus on reactivating dormant parts of the brain not only can we create lives that we are more than happy with, we can actually start to change the way the DNA is read over the succeeding generation to move towards our original blueprint.

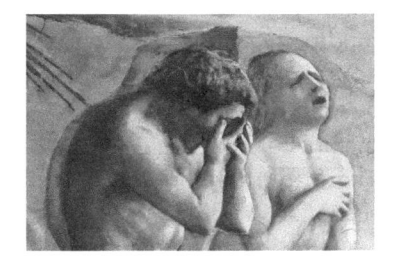

John Lash, comparative mythologist and author of "Not In his Image" promotes the power of myth to change human destiny. When he discovered the Sophia Myth, the sacred story of the earth's dreaming he knew he had found something that stood out beyond other myths. It is the most suppressed mythology we know of today.

When we place our lives and life stories within the bigger story of humanity, that of the Earth, Gaia Sophia and life itself, something very magical starts to happen, we gain a sense of direction and meaning and the mundane matters of every day affairs come to life. Gnostic mythology, rediscovered through John Lash's work with the Nag Hammadi Scrolls and telestic methods tells of human degeneration and disconnection from nature, the Earth and source, a gender rift and a fall into patriarchal belief systems. Through learning and living within the story we can generate a storyline whereby we get back on track.
You can find further material regarding this chapter at:

Return to the Brain of Eden by Tony Wright and Graham Gynn
Not in His Image by John Lash
foodforconsciousness.blogspot.com
leftinthedark.org.uk
beyond-belief.org.uk
metahistory.org
There are more references in the Appendices of this book and references section.

3. Getting Back on Track of your True Peak Potential

In this chapter we set out in the quest for our most exalted possible state, where we feel and function at our best. I describe three areas to focus on, which weave together to take us on our way. There are many things we can do to move into a more enjoyable and functional state of being quite quickly. Over time we can experience more substantial improvement, while major changes are possible for succeeding generations. We now move into the practical. Consistency gives the best results when making practical changes. It doesn't matter if we fall off the wagon from time to time – that's understandable – the most important thing is that we pick ourselves up and get on with something constructive again.

Gradual changes that we stick with and build up are worth more than flash in the pan experiments that we leave behind. Also they are more doable. As our brain chemistry and sense of self shifts we act from a different place, our world changes for the better, and it's easier to do a bit more. Along the way we may well meet resistance and challenges as we move from one set of perceptions about life to another but as we work through them life gets more satisfying at a deeper, less shakeable level. The most painful thing we can do in life is not to live to our true purpose and potential. Living our purpose connects us with the life force and gives us energy we would not otherwise have.

With the necessary nutrients and hormones in place from before conception, children could potentially be born with full perception and function in both hemispheres and a whole sense of self. For those of us already born, again with the necessary nutrients and hormones, the left hemisphere stranglehold significantly lessened, and with skilful lifestyle practices, we still have the capacity for genius abilities. We can live in profound connection at a feeling level with nature and our environment, have complete empathy with each other, live in harmony with everything around us, and experience phenomenal pleasure from these simple things.

In days of antiquity the human situation was better understood. It was known that we were slipping into a decline and measures were put in place to help. Treatments for the condition have been handed down to us in the form of the various traditional spiritual and shamanic practices. Many of them are still helpful but, by themselves, they are not enough to heal or reverse the condition. We are now in a situation where we have technology to assist us and this has allowed the information revolution so that knowledge of the human condition and the remedies is becoming available With our natural abilities restored we would not be so reliant on the technology that got us towards the fix. It's a heartening thought.

What is potentially available to us?

"If we can recreate our ancestral hormonal environment through diet and a sustained reversal of cerebral dominance, a very different human may emerge. One with enhanced perception, a stronger immune system, more balanced dexterity, more efficient digestion and greater physical and mental capability. We would experience more profound and pleasurable sexuality too, coupled with a reproductive system that works as intended. Even baldness would no longer be a problem. Most crucially, society would become much less aggressive and violent because our sense of self would change radically. Such a restoration of consciousness, with all these attendant benefits, is more that a theoretical possibility." Tony Wright.

Potentially available to all of us are genius abilities – and also the capacity for deep bliss. At present our powers of creative consciousness are largely kept literally at a dream level. The more conscious we become the greater our ability to manifest our greatest dreams. Humans whose brains were fully connected would feel an automatic empathy with each other and their environment and would create a happier and more harmonious world.

What might we be able to gain from the research into the exalted states of consciousness that some have glimpses of:

Biological - enhanced immune system, fully functioning gut therefore increased assimilation, clearer vision, sharper hearing, enhanced taste, better skin tone, stronger leaner muscles, correct weight, clean systems, fully functioning organs. Enhanced neural system enhances health.

Connection - feelings of oneness and bliss, connection to all living things, connection to sacred earth energy spots, and nature in general, psychic abilities, being able to travel out of body, telepathy. Feeling fulfilled even in the face of life's challenges, a feeling of being at home in ourselves and connected to something larger.

Intellectual - genius abilities in all academic ability - maths, language, science, artistic, musical etc

Social - social harmony, social responsibility, social empathy

Longevity - we are developing neurally and mentally, until at least our fifties and almost certainly beyond. We are not designed to age as fast as we do. The causes of our premature ageing are to be found in our environment, internal hormonal environment and damage to parts of the DNA through our lives. The trigger point for accelerated ageing is the hormonal change at puberty. If you think about it a child in late adolescence can be very grown up and capable, but they are not ageing. They are also incredible good at learning, they have neuroplasticity. There are a lot of clues here and we come back to this topic in chapter 9.

There are three strands to human correction which weave together, but it's easier to approach them one by one. The physical, the mental and connection.

Physical

Our observations and choices at the physical and material level. Physiology and posture, natural nutrition and lifestyle. This includes nourishing and rebuilding the neural system, and activating it which is why I often call it neuroactive nutrition. It has the effects of optimising bodily health too, and also beginning to read the DNA in a more favourable way.

Mental

Reengaging the true imagination, making choices in mental realm, the use of language, reclaiming your mind from cultural conditioning. Focusing on true healthy desires, living the real dream of your life, reactivating the dormant right hemisphere with all it's creativity and enhanced faculties, regaining a sense of peace with the world.

"Nirvana is what you see now liberated from any conceptual elaborations" John Lash

Connection

Harmonious connection with each other, nature, plant realms, animal relatives, the Earth, the Stars and Source. Natural lifestyle. Mirroring attention. The quest for the Grail, the Organic Light, and living in the sacred narrative. Healing of the gender rift. Less disparity between people of different ages.

Paradise on Earth

When we do our part, our biological habitat the Earth adjusts to make paradise for us. This is a mystery that we do not need to understand but does indeed come true. It's quite speculative for me but I remember when other topics in this book where equally mysterious to me so I keep an open mind. A simple example of the kind of thing that nature can do is the way mushrooms have eaten up radioactive contaminants inside the old reactors at Chernobyl. The problems created in Earth are too big for us to solve, especially from our current state of awareness. Our focus needs to be on recovering our humanity, in connection with benign forces much larger than us.

When I found the answer to the question in my mind of what has happened to us as humans in terms of the biochemistry and so forth I wondered how we could proceed. For sure this knowledge needs to be spread and action taken, but a collective solution presents problems. To abandon our lives for a cause would be to miss the point, because our aim is to reach our full potential as humans, not to sacrifice our lives. I concluded that the best way forward would be to bring together what I have learned and present it as a kind of recipe for individual fulfilment. In the words of John Lash "You do not live for humanity but it can live through you when you hold to the solidarity of the Anthropos, that luminous child" . (The Anthropos is a name for the human species, in the same way as feline is a name for the cat species, or canine for the dog species). While humans love to help each other, service in the form of sacrifice is a not a natural part of our make up, it's a later part of cultural conditioning. Sacrificing our happiness to others cannot be an ideal because if everyone did it everyone would be unhappy. We are here to live our unique life potentials to the full and inspire others to do the same. In the words of Howard Thurman, "Don't ask what the world needs. Ask what makes you come alive, and go do it. Because what the world needs is people who have come alive."

Fractal rather than 'viral' is the natural organic way that knowledge is transmitted. In a fractal, although each newly generated part is similar it is not necessarily an exact replica. This is generation not cloning. Fractality is aligned with the Fibonacci system of numbers. Each successive number is a created by adding the two that precede it. 1, 1, 2, 3, 5, 8, 13, 21, 34, 55 and so on. In this means of spreading knowledge there is person 1, who imparts to another person 2, so we have two people. Person 1 shares with person 3, then we have three people.. Person 1 and person 2 each share again, bringing the total to 5. The first three then share again making the total 8. And so it goes on. Very quickly a large number of people are involved, knowledge I spreading. If the original participants are still l active, and sharing their ideas and energy they are growing and diversifying through new people.. Of course if a few drop out, it does not stymie the progress of the whole thing. This is an organic process, growing rather than spreading like an illness. The problems that humanity faces could be more aptly viewed as spread by a virus, a virus of ideas and philosophies, of programming that are actually foreign and invasive to human nature. The solution is fractal. The knowledge is spread energetically and experientally, as well as conceptually, in the spirit of kindness and friendship rather than righteousness. That's why it is better done in person.

We can get started right away. Whatever situation we are in there are certain things we have control of. From there we can manage ourselves and expand the improvement in our lives. The times we live in are challenging and full of conflict. We are not in a Golden age, but we can glimpses of the next one emerging and live partly in it. Knowing that we are at this juncture, where humanity is challenged so deeply and the odds are so high, can spur us on to a deeply satisfying life where we can make a big beneficial difference. We can live heroic lives of enormous fulfilment, on an epic journey, with an epic storyline with many themes, adventure, romance in the true sense, beauty and humour. We need to take care not to get lost in the details of the microcosm and the personal dramas but keep our heads high and connected to the macrocosm, the bigger picture. The life force is stronger than any other force in our lives.

A wonderful instant way to change state is described by Tony Robbins as The Triad. It consists of three actions. They are changing your posture, changing the language you use and changing what you are focusing on. Something I really like about is that it is an instant starting point for the three part correction, because it uses physiology, language and focus. Once we are in a more positive state it's easier to start putting into place ongoing measures to move into a more permanently improved state.

In the next chapter I begin looking at our physiological state with talking about how we can return to our natural biological diet as humans. Of course this inevitably affects our mental state and our sense of connection. Finding our authentic sense of self, breaking out of programming and living a true ever unfolding life story is a fabulous contribution we can make and the best life we know of.

4. Eating the Biological Diet of Our Species

Learning about natural nutrition is just which nutritional components we take in. It is also about getting into states of mind where we can trust our intuition about what to eat. The nutrition in this book is aimed to get us into our natural intuitive waking dream state where we can live the lives we truly want to live and intuitively know what we need to eat. It is when we have gone off track that we need some guidance to get back into it. That is the situation most of us find ourselves in within our culture.

I did not know all the components of the biological diet when I began so it was not all smooth sailing. In spite of this it was a total revelation to me how the way we eat affects the way we feel and function. My starting point was moving to a completely raw food diet of raw fruits, vegetables, soaked seeds, cold pressed oils and a few other additions such as raw miso. After about 72 hours I felt myself move into a noticeably different state, one that has been described as the 'raw high'. I felt like a child in the garden, in a flow, life felt like a song and my intuition was sky high. I knew just what I had to do, from the little practical details of life, to the bigger projects. I felt extraordinarily energised and found I needed two hours less sleep a night and the sleep I had felt more refreshing. It felt like there was more intelligent connection between my waking and sleeping states. In short my quality of life was radically improved.

There are so many beneficial changes experienced by many people on this path. I list them later in this chapter. I was intrigued to know what it is about this way of eating that has such an impact. I wanted to know how I could take it further and how to make it work nutritionally. You now have the benefit of what I learned without having to go through the detective trail I did! You can make any adaptations you need for your individual circumstances. You don't need to eat all your food raw although I highly recommend eating predominantly raw foods to get the maximum out of your life; and I recommend selecting your cooked foods with care. I go through this in chapter 2.

I feel that sometimes people would like to just circumnavigate the step of optimising their nutrition. Changing what we eat is a huge thing to do. Eating habits are hardwired into us in infancy, and our cultural identity and social lives are tied up with them. Many foods are even addictive. Replacing our cultural eating patterns is in some ways very hard, and in some ways surprisingly easy once you take the plunge. I wish it could be true that you could just 'think different thoughts' and it won't matter what you eat. The simple fact is that unless you nourish and fuel your neural system the way it was designed to be, you will never experience the full potential of what you might be and do.

Sometimes people say that the world's problems can be solved with love. This could be true in a roundabout way. Until we have the neural capacity to feel and have empathy then love remains a concept or dogma. As Tony Wright puts it it's like a hare telling a tortoise 'all you have to do is run faster'. Without the anatomical capacity that is wish rather than a plan.

In an age when the knowledge of biological diet is becoming more and more widespread, implementing it is already becoming a trend, especially amongst the youngest generation. These people are giving themselves enormous advantages in every area of life. With the increasing challenges we face in the world many people are concluding that this is a choice that they cannot afford not to make. On the bright side, because of this it becomes easier and easier to do. There are not many places now where you cannot get a salad or fruit; superfoods and supplements are very easy to obtain and really the world is now laid out for us to enjoy and embrace this lifestyle.

My original aim which led me to this way of eating was a simple desire to feel good and experience an expanded sense of connection. All these years later I find that the nutritional recommendations for avoiding degenerative disease are along the same lines. If we want our health and sense of youthfulness long term we need to commit to nature's way, the ways of the planet we inhabit. This is a simple fact of life.

This chapter gives a comprehensive description of the kinds of foods that are ideal for humans to eat in order to satisfy our nutritional needs, taking account of the complexities of the situation we are in. It does not come from a dogmatic point of view, rather a mechanical or biological view of what we actually need to function and feel at our best, based on the experience of many people over a long time. We are all individuals with slight variations in our needs, but the essentials are pretty much the same for all of us.

We can move towards the nutrient rich plant based raw diet that is natural to our species. It's truly a miracle that we can build human beings out of pastry and pasta, but we will never feel our best on it. The need to adapt back to a natural diet is a big challenge for many people. Commitment and being willing to venture out of our current comfort zones is required. The rest of what we need to do is actually a lot easier. Changing what we eat is a matter of adjusting to a different way of going about things and a new range of tastes. Most people soon report on how much better they feel AND how much more pleasurable food becomes. Once the change is made it is actually easier than the old way. One of the main purposes of this book is to make it easier and more fun – and get the nutrition sustainable.

I have looked at our original human biological diet which enhanced our neural function and experience of life so much, considered what has happened to us and where we are now, and brought in the commonalities found in all healthy groups by Weston Price. The aim is to keep it light enough to feel that natural high and cognitive ecstasy, while dense enough to nourish us long term. We can put together a way of eating that covers all these commonalities for physical strength and health in a way that optimises our chances for taking ourselves to the next level in the way we feel and function. In the West now we have access to foods from round the world and can obtain in our biological foods even if we live a long way from where they are grown. This way of eating is by necessity a mix of compromises because we are in a compromised situation.

What are the nutritional components we need?

In order to build and fuel our neural system to full capacity we need adequate amounts of undamaged fatty acids, undamaged amino acids and undamaged fruit compounds (flavonoids) plus a myriad of other plant compounds. We also need the basic elements of matter known as minerals. In this section I expand on this and the general nutrition we need for well-being.

The basic elements our bodies are made of are minerals. We cannot make these in our own bodies nor can plants or animals make them. The need to be present in the soil that plants grow in so that the plants can turn them into a form that we can assimilate them in. Some of these minerals such as magnesium and sulphur we need in comparatively large quantities. Others, the trace minerals, we need in tiny amounts but these tiny amounts are crucial to the running of our bodies and brains. Altogether we need over 60 minerals for proper functioning.

Now we come to the compounds or chemical structures that are made of minerals. Please bear with me if you are a chemistry expert. I know there are readers who appreciate this clarification. We also need about 16 vitamins to get these mineral elements to where they need to be. These can be manufactured by plants from the basic mineral elements. From plants we also need a huge variety of compounds such as flavonoids which act as antioxidants, mono amine oxidase inhibitors and so forth.

We need amino acids, the building blocks of proteins to build tissues, generate neurotransmitters, make enzymes and more. Those amino acids we cannot make within our own bodies we call essential amino acids and there are eight to twelve of them depending on our ability to manufacture one amino acid from another.

We need various fatty acids to build and insulate neural tissue amongst other things. Those we cannot make ourselves in our bodies are called essential fatty acids. The polyunsaturated fats omega 3 (linolenic) and omega 6 (linoleic) fatty acids and omega 9 (monounsaturated) fatty acids are in this group.

Ideally we take in all these nutritional components in undamaged form, i.e. not heated above biological temperature.

This is the basic list of the nutrients we know we need not counting the myriad of plant compounds and cofactors that we do not yet fully understand.

Essential minerals

Almost 99% of the mass of the human body is made up of six elements: oxygen, carbon, hydrogen, nitrogen, calcium, and phosphorus. About 0.85% is composed of another five elements: potassium, sulphur, sodium, chlorine, and magnesium. All 11 are necessary for life. There are sixty plus other minerals which are needed in small amounts and are necessary of power bodily function. Some of them are: cobalt, copper, aluminium, arsenic, barium, beryllium, boron, bromine, iodine, iron, manganese, selenium, zinc, cerium, caesium, chromium, dysprosium, erbium, europium, gadolinium, gallium, germanium, gold, hafnium, holmium, lanthanum, lithium, lutetium, molybdenum, neodymium, nickel, niobium, praseodymium, rhenium, rubidium, samarium, scandium, silicon, silver, strontium, tantalum, terbium, thulium, tin, titanium, vanadium, ytterbium, yttrium, and zirconium

We are used to hearing about deforestation in the Amazon but it's easily forgotten that even Europe was once densely forested. With the loss of forest came loss of soil quality and loss of essential nutrients in the soil. Industrial agriculture since the second world war has added to the damage. The practice of harvesting the land for food without replacing what is taken from the soil by recycling organic waste means that, for most of us, our food today has far less mineral content than it did even a few decades ago. NPK farming, introduced in the twentieth century is farming using fertilisers containing nitrogen, phosphorus and potassium. These minerals will enable the plants to grow well but will not enable them to provide all the minerals we need to flourish.

I feel to emphasise again that minerals are the basic building blocks. They are not made by us or by plants, they come from the Earth itself. If we cannot take them in through food then we need to supplement one way or another.

Some of the minerals that are most likely to be seriously deficient include sulphur, zinc, iodine, selenium, magnesium, chromium, silicon and iron for young women and children. To find out which minerals you may be lacking it is a good idea to get a mineral test done. You may be amazed at what minerals you are lacking and how much that explains about your health and food cravings.

Obviously we take in oxygen through breathing and water gives us hydrogen and oxygen. Carbon is in our foods in carbohydrates, fats and amino acids (protein). Nitrogen is in amino acids. The remaining minerals need also to be replenished through food or supplementation and in a useable form. If we look at the list of minerals we need we can see how we can easily have serious deficiencies in magnesium and sulphur and may need relatively high supplementation of these two minerals. Calcium can potentially be an issue too. Then we need also the so-called trace elements, those we need but only in tiny quantities.

In mineral extensive mineral testing I observed that most people are lacking in sulphur, magnesium, silicon and chromium. Many are also lacking iodine, zinc and selenium. To compound the problem there are so many toxic elements in the environment now including large amounts of aluminium that nearly everyone is overloaded with them. Aluminium binds with sulphur and silicon. Supplementing judiciously with sulphur can help to flush out toxic elements and also improve sulphur levels. Then when supplementing with silicon the body can use it rather than it being bound up with aluminium. Magnesium needs to be added in supplemental form for most people. A good trace mineral supplement is also necessary. Sulphur is best taken in the form of organic MSM, stirred into water and thirty minutes before any other supplement or food. Chromium is essential for sugar metabolism. A deficiency can cause carbohydrate cravings and ultimately lead to diabetes. By the way an apparent phosphorus deficiency can indicate lack of vitamin C. Not only are our diets deficient but we are dealing with environmental toxicity and vitamin C is one of our first lines of defence.

Essential Vitamins

Vitamin A, Vitamin B1 (Thiamine,) Vitamin B2 (Riboflavin), Vitamin B3 (Niacin), Vitamin B5 (Pantothenic Acid), Vitamin B6 (Pyridoxine), Vitamin B7 (biotin), Vitamin B9 (folic acid), Vitamin B12 (Cobalamin), Vitamin C, Vitamin D3, Vitamin E,Vitamin K, Choline, Flavonoids and Bioflavonoids, Inositol

Essential Amino Acids

Valine, Lysine, Threonine, Leucine, Isoleucine, Tryptophan, Phenylalanine,, Methionine, Histidine, Arginine, Taurine, Tyrosine

In the diet these amino acids can come from many sources. In plant based diets we need to take care that we take in all the essential amino acids. Plant foods contain protein for sure but protein just means a combination of amino acids . We need to include these specific amino acids. This can be done, it just takes sone thought. Traditional vegetarian diets take it into account.

Essential Fatty Acids: Omega 3 (EPA, DHA, ALA), Omega 6, Omega 9
These can obtained mostly from cold pressed seed oils and butters, blended soaked seeds, nuts (in moderation) olive oil and coconut oil. DHA and EPA I explain later.

Pineal Biochemicals

In addition to all this are the botanicals which compensate for the biochemicals we have lost due to the under function of the thyroid gland. The biochemicals include melatonin, DMT in tiny amounts, and pinoline, a mono amine oxidase inhibitor.

Why Raw Food ?

In our natural habitat our biological foods were eaten naturally without cooking, there simply was so need or desire to change them in this way. Cooking came later as a survival strategy.

Eating predominantly raw natural food gives a feeling that's almost impossible to describe. It brings a connection to the forces of nature that protects us from the unwanted stimuli and messages of the artificial world. It strengthens the mind in its connection to the life force and hones the intuition to guide us through safely, happily and in alignment with our destiny. It connects us through living fractal structure to resources beyond or normal senses. It places you in the living matrix, a profoundly different paradigm to that constructed by the limited left hemisphere. It connects us to the Earth in a real felt sense. That's why more can be learned about it through the experience than a description of that experience. It's why actually doing it consistently is the way to learn about it.

People experience a myriad of benefits from eating their food predominantly raw: increased energy, less need for sleep, improvement in general health, uplifted mood, ideal weight, shining eyes, beautiful skin, younger looks, clearer thinking and intuition, enhanced creativity, increased effectiveness, calmer and more contented children and heightened physical sensations. Many people notice that their connections to nature and to other people deepen and they gain what can be described as a more spiritual and sensual experience of life. On a lighter note many people also find that when they eat a clean diet and consume a large amount of raw fruit and vegetables, their skin colour changes to a richer colour and their skin responds differently to sun, tanning rather than burning.

Why is this?

Firstly it clears out toxic sludge that the body simply does not know what to do with. Secondly it rebuilds the neural system with the construction materials it was designed to be built with. Thirdly it provides the ideal fuel. Fourthly it contains powerful biochemicals that naturally modulate our neural chemistry. Fifthly we are on our way to our DNA being read a little more optimally.

Heating above body temperature changes the molecular structure of food. The nutrients in uncooked food are in a form that the body can recognise, understand and use. Food in its natural living state has a crystalline structure with electromagnetic fields which carry order and information into the body and brain. In particular, a balanced, fresh, nutrient rich diet provides undamaged amino acids, fatty acids and fruit compounds such as flavonoids.

After water, the main constituent of the brain is fat. As already mentioned, the nerve membranes and insulating myelin sheaths are made of fatty acids (fats) and it is important that we consume a good range of undamaged (raw, unprocessed) healthy fats to give these parts of the brain their correct structure. The fatty acids in our brain are extremely delicate and prone to oxidative damage. In nature they are always wrapped up with antioxidants. Immersion in antioxidant compounds thus protects our brains. Undamaged or raw means not heated above biological temperature, above which the molecules are deranged. This is approximately body temperature.

The neurotransmitters in our brains are generally a class of biochemicals called monoamines and they are constructed from amino acids, the substances of which proteins are made. The undamaged nature of raw amino acids improves neurotransmitter quality.

The mono-amine oxidase inhibiting effects of the flavonoids in fruit and in various other foods and herbs help keep the neurotransmitter levels high. These in turn stimulate the pineal gland and the production of even more powerful pineal monoamine oxidase inhibitors (MAOI's), which further boost neuroactivity. Tryptophan, one of the essential amino acids that we need to consume because it is not made inside the body, is the amino acid most damaged by heating. Cooked diets inevitably lower tryptophan levels. As serotonin and melatonin are made from tryptophan this has a deleterious effect on mood and sense of well-being.

Food in its raw, undamaged state, is something the body can easily process. Removing cooked food, especially cooked fats and proteins, removes the sludge that the body does not know what to do with leaving us feeling clearer and with less blockage to the energy of life.

Moving from the biological slant to a more esoteric and geometrical one, the structure of all living things is intricately based on the golden ratio or phi. This structure lends itself to life, growth, movement, connection and, in a word, fractality. Nature - from the cosmic to the biological to the microscopic - is fractal. If you take any small part of it you can build the whole thing from the information contained in it. For example the DNA blueprint for construction of the whole human body is in every cell of the body. The more we surround ourselves and fill ourselves with living matter, the more we keep ourselves in touch with that all powerful, all knowing, ever present fractal reality or 'divine' or natural intelligence and awareness. Used in art and music, the golden ratio is pleasing to the eye and the ear. It gives us a sense of beauty and pleasure and natural things are the ultimate pleasure. Because the structure of raw food has not been changed on a molecular level by heating it retains more fractality. The integrity of the fractal patterning is even greater in some raw foods than others for example natural wild foods and hemp - their structure allows us to connect better with the universal 'divine' fractal pattern. This sense of connection could be seen as the essence of the 'spiritual' experience, that indefinable expansion of energy and awareness, and it is so more easily felt in natural surroundings and sacred places where that patterning is much more intact. Perhaps the right hemisphere of the brain has retained a greater capability to align with fractal reality. Entheagenic nutrition is another way to describe our biological diet. Entheogenic means generating a sense of the divine within.

Put another way, natural raw food connects us to the Earth. It's very noticeable, especially when you forage greens or pick your own fruits, that you form a perceptible connection to the tree or land where your food came from.

'Spiritual awareness' is inherently connected to physical awareness – they are both energetic awareness. With increased energetic awareness our vision, hearing, smell, taste and touch senses become more sensitive and accurate too. Psychic, supernatural and physical senses only seem separate to us because we use a different of our minds to access to access information beyond the limited level of five sense sensations that are currently the usual experience. When we go into that different part of our minds (the right hemisphere it would seem from research) we perceive and feel different and experience a different sense of self which feels very profound. Obviously there are many tools used to access this part of ourselves – high quality living food gives us good building blocks to lay a foundation for increased sensitivity.

Raw food is utterly delicious. Interestingly, after some time on a raw diet most people prefer the natural tastes. But even before that adaptation, beautiful raw recipe creations can be made which taste as good as cooked. What's more, the increased sensitivity we begin to acquire gives us an eating experience which is sensual on a different level – every mouthful becomes exquisite. The tastes and colours of the food are more vibrant making a wonderful cuisine out of entirely healthy ingredients. It is hardly surprising that the natural diet of our species is also delicious to us.

For long term health many experts agree that it's best to eat at least 50% of your food raw. I would say as high a percentage as you can to feel the benefits I have described. The five fruit and vegetable a day rule could be more sensibly replaced by something like 25 or more, at least some of it blended to do some of the work that once our digestive system could do. Personally I find to eat nearly all raw but allowing myself hot drinks is a great compromise, the raw high with the comfort of warmth and the option of teas and and herbal drinks. After you have read what I am about to write you too might decide that you too want to stick to raw foods as much as you can. I am going to talk here about problems of cooked foods too as well as extolling the virtues of raw foods because I think it's important to understand how alien cooked food ultimately is to us, even though there may be a time and place for its use in the situation we are currently in. After eating primarily raw foods for a while, with only carefully selected cooked foods included if any, the experience of eating heavy cooked food can be akin to getting drunk, with even a mild hangover the next day. A sobering thought!

Digestive leukocytosis is an increase in white blood cells occurring after eating cooked food, indicating that the body is responding to an attack. It does not occur after eating raw food. In 1930, under the direction of Dr. Paul Kouchakoff, research was conducted at the Institute of Clinical Chemistry in Lausanne, Switzerland. The effect of food on the immune system was tested and documented. They found that after eating cooked food a human's blood responds immediately by increasing the number of white blood cells. Since this digestive leukocytosis was always observed after a meal, it was considered to be a normal physiological response to eating. No one knew why the number of white cells rises after eating, since this appeared to be a stress response; as if the body was somehow reacting to something harmful, in the way it would react to an infection.

It was then found that eating raw, unaltered food did not cause a reaction in the blood. In addition, they found that if a food had been heated beyond a certain temperature (which is unique to each food) or if the food was processed, refined or had chemicals added, this always caused a rise in the number of white cells in the blood. The researchers renamed this reaction 'pathological leukocytosis', since the body was reacting to altered food.

Now onto Maillard's molecules. These are chemicals created when food is heated to high temperatures above about 130 degrees Celsius in the absence of moisture. This happens particularly in baking, frying. grilling or roasting. These chemicals are created by amino acids (proteins) and sugars (such as fructose and glucose) when they are heated together. They are what gives cooked food its browned appearance. Maillard reactions were first described by a French physician and biochemist, Louis-Camille Maillard, in 1912. These reactions produce hundreds of chemical compounds that give colour and aroma to many of the foods people love, but the chemicals are actually toxic to us. Foods cooked by boiling or steaming do not turn brown or acquire the complexity of flavours because the temperature only reaches about 100°C.

Acrylamides formed in cooked carbohydrates came to public attention in 2002 when Swedish officials were so alarmed by recent research findings that they decided to inform the public immediately rather than wait for them to be published in a scientific journal. Shortly afterwards, the World Health Organization held a three-week emergency meeting to evaluate the Swedish scientists' recent discovery. They learned that starchy foods, such as potato chips, french fries, baked potatoes, biscuits and bread, contain very high levels of acrylamides, chemicals that have been shown to cause genetic mutations leading to a range of cancers in rats. Acrylamides are considered 1,000 times more dangerous than the majority of cancer-causing agents found in food. They have been found to cause benign and malignant stomach tumours, as well as damage to the central and peripheral nervous system. The safe levels for acrylamides has been set at zero by the US Environmental Protection Agency yet they continue to be eaten in every day foods.

In addition, cooked carbohydrates contain glycotoxins, including advanced glycation end products (AGE's). The May 2003 edition of Life Extension magazine discusses AGEs, referring to a new study published in the Proceedings of the National Academy of Sciences. Advanced glycation end products are proteins or lipids that become glycated as a result of exposure to sugars. Eating food cooked at high temperatures causes the formation of AGEs, which accelerate ageing. AGEs also cause chronic inflammation, which can lead to devastating, even lethal, effects directly involved with diseases like diabetes, cancer, atherosclerosis, congestive heart failure, aortic valve stenosis, Alzheimer's and kidney impairment.

When you heat protein to very high temperatures you get a carcinogenic by-product called heterocyclic amines. Quoting the article above "Cooking and ageing have similar biological properties. The process that turns a broiled chicken brown illustrates what happens to our body's proteins as we age. As the proteins react with sugars, they turn brown and lose elasticity; they cross-link to form insoluble masses that generate free radicals (which contribute to ageing). The resulting AGEs accumulate in our collagen, skin, cornea of the eye, brain, nervous system, vital organs and arteries as we age. Normal ageing can also be regarded as a slow cooking process." The glycation reaction cross-links the body's proteins, making them barely functional. Their accumulation causes cells to emit signals that produce dangerous inflammation.

Research at the Max Planck Institute for National Research in Germany shows that coagulation of proteins by cooking makes them only half as assimilable. The change in the molecular structure of the proteins make cellular healing, reproduction and regeneration difficult. Up to 50% of cooked proteins that one eats will coagulate and cross-link. Heating protein above 104° F (40° C) begins to produce toxins. Higher temperatures create even more dangerous toxins, such as heterocyclic amines (HCAs), which are caustic compounds that have proven to cause cancer in laboratory animals. Some HCAs are so toxic to the neurotransmitters and their receptors in the brain that they eventually cause brain diseases, such as Alzheimer's, Parkinson's and schizophrenia.

Fats heated above 96° F (36° C) create lipid peroxides, which are oily, oxidizing compounds, proven carcinogens. Heating unsaturated fats (polyunsaturated and monounsaturated fats i.e., those liquid at room temperature in temperate zones, at high heat produces trans fatty acids, which create toxic free radicals in the body that cause cancer, ageing and liver toxicity. Heated oils also contain mycotoxins.

The story of Pottenger's cats is interesting. Between 1932 and 1942, Dr Pottenger conducted a clinical trial, involving over nine hundred cats over nine generations, into the nutritional effects of cooked versus raw food diets. Group one was fed raw meat scraps including organ meats and bone, and raw milk. Group two was fed the same scraps but cooked, and were given pasteurised (heat treated) milk. The cats on raw food were healthy, averaged five kittens per litter with few birthing problems, and most died of old age. After nine generations there was no change in their health status.

The cats in group two however began developing problems from the first generation, with increased deaths in the litters, smaller litter sizes, poorer mothering, noticeable dull rough coats. From the second generation onwards there were vision problems which were probably taurine deficiency, common infections, and dermatitis, arthritis, heart disease (taurine again), allergies, gingivitis and periodontal disease, inflamed joints and nervous tissue, and skeletal malformation. Fertility and litter size declined rapidly, and perinatal mortality increased. Behaviourally the group on cooked food became progressively more aggressive to handlers and each other. Gastrointestinal parasitism was a major problem in the cooked food group but not the raw food group. By the fifth generation on cooked food the cats were completely sterile and had stopped reproducing.

Pottenger found that by changing the diet from cooked back to raw he could reverse most of the symptoms, but only until early in the third generation. From the fourth generation onwards much of the damage was irreversible. This suggests that damage from a cooked food diet has a generationally compounding effect. He repeated the experiment on white mice and got similar results.

Clearly we are not cats, but still the question begs to be asked - how many generations of people will there be living in cities away from nature and eating junk food?

Cooked Foods to include and not include

We have seen how cooking was an invention that allowed us to eat foods that grow outside our natural biological habitat and how cooked foods can still fill nutritional gaps today in the foods we have available. We have seen that we also need to take great care in the way we go about it, There are some foods that are not natural to us that actually should not be eaten in large quantities raw but instead fermented as a first preference or cooked. For example the cruciferous vegetables such as kale, spinach, cabbage, cauliflower and broccoli contain substances called goitrogens which inhibit iodine uptake by the the thyroid. Eating large amounts of them raw over a period of time can affect thyroid function. Cooking or fermenting them breaks down the goitrogens. Then of course there are foods such as beans and rice which can fill in protein and B vitamin gaps if we choose to do it that way. These can be fermented after cooking so we get products such as miso. Unpasteurised miso could be described as a living food even though it is not technically raw as it has been brought to life by microorganisms.

We are going to feel better if we keep these cooked foods to a minimum. As we have seen, cooked proteins do not have the same pristine quality as undamaged uncooked ones. We need to be careful with cooked and processed fats too. Saturated fats, in particular coconut oil, are the best to use for cooking because they are stable when heated. Polyunsaturated fats such as seed oils and monounsaturated fats such as olive oil are unstable in the presence of heat, light and air and need to be kept sealed and cool and definitely not used for cooking. When these fats are heated their molecular structure changes and they become foreign sludge in our bodies. Butter and ghee are also saturated fats and are the second best choice after coconut oil for any cooking we may choose to do.

Other reasons we may want to eat cooked food at times are social. At informal gatherings it's easy to make delicious raw recipes that others will love, but sometimes there are occasions where this is not so possible or appropriate. What we want to avoid is a massive loss of energy after eating supercharged nutrition for a while. It's easy to take this level of energy for granted after while and organise our lives accordingly. For all these reasons I provide a list of foods that are beneficial cooked. And I provide another list of cooked foods to avoid altogether because of the health problems and mood drops they cause.

Cooked foods that may be helpful at times and do not cause too many problems include natural corn, rice, beans such as black beans, steamed winter vegetables, coconut oil, herbal teas and some herbs that are more effective when heat treated.

Foods to definitely avoid include:
- Refined sugar. This has a negative effect on the immune system and metabolism. It also depletes mineral levels and feeds degenerative diseases. Of course it excess it leads to metabolic disorders.
- Grains. According to the noted expert on this subject, Dr Peter Osborne, the number one thing you can do to overcome autoimmune disorders is to remove grains from your diet. Gluten, by definition, is the family of proteins found in the seeds of grasses. There are many types of gluten. These proteins are at best not ideal for humans and at worst lead to degenerative disease. Mood swings, gut problems and appetite disorders are other common reactions. Gluten is a neurotoxin. How much grain consumption you choose may depend on your individual sensitivity and also the level of well-being you want to achieve. Some people who stop eating them for a while can even feel drunk on trying them again.
- A1 type milk from modern breeds of cows (see next section).
- Soy. Soy inhibits the conversion of tyrosine into essential neurotransmitters. It suppresses the thyroid gland. In cultures

that traditionally used soy beans they were mostly fermented and only small amounts used. At this level soy can have benefits. Avoid large quantities of soy, especially if it is unfermented.

Processed and heated oils and proteins I have mentioned.

Various allergenic foods. For some people peanuts, eggs, tomatoes, peppers and aubergines are problematic. It is great idea to have in depth allergy testing because apparently healthy foods that are good for most people may cause reactions in a few individuals. There may even be delayed reactions that we don't notice but could undermine our health long term.

Whys and Why Nots of Eating Animal Foods

We can survive on existing reserves of some nutrients for a long while as adults, but when they are diminished enough we will notice a change in how we feel. When I discovered the benefits of raw food I took it for granted that I would be sticking to raw plant foods. The benefits and increase in energy I experienced were so wonderful that I wanted to continue like this. When, after a period of time, I became malnourished I realised what nutrients I had been missing. I had symptoms of deficiency of vitamin D even though I was supplementing this vitamin and also vitamin A in the form of retinol, and protein even though I was eating seeds. Through researching further and talking to many people about their experiences I came to the conclusion that long term it works out better to include either some cooked foods or some animal products which can be vegetarian options such as milk products.

How can cooked foods make a difference? For one thing it increases options. For example some people include fortified foods that contain the vitamins missing from plant foods such as A, D and B vitamins especially B12. Also, on the protein front, cooked food combinations such as beans and other pulses and rice, which although not original biological foods any more than cheese is, are an inventive way of obtaining those pieces of nutrition that we would have automatically got in the forest. It's another way of obtaining all the nutrients we need to survive and covering the commonalities that I describe in the next section about Dr Weston Price.

Over centuries cultures have worked out ways to meet nutritional needs. And while we set out on this new path we would be wise to take note. Although it is sometimes said we don't need that much protein this is a bit of a reaction to the excess meat consumption of some modern cultures. The truth is all body growth and replacement needs protein or in fact the amino acids that make it up. Also, many of our neurotransmitters are made from amino acids. Personally I prefer to eat as much of my food raw as possible and eat raw cheese and kefir. But I also see high raw diets with supplementation and strategically chosen cooked foods working well long term too.

Insects, or their material, within fruits were part of our original diet and did provide essential nutrients for our needs. We do need a source of these nutrients. The fruit we generally find to eat today in civilisation really has a quite different nutritional profile. Traditional cultures consume some sort of animal protein and fat from fish and other seafood, water and land fowl, land animals, eggs, milk and milk products, reptiles, and insects.

What can we use in our modern forest diet? Each person has their view on the ethical issues. Personally my own ethic is that restoring human consciousness is a priority for the sake of every species on the planet and this includes adequate human nutrition. All animal species will prioritise their own nutritional needs and especially those of their young. If you the reader are one of those growing numbers of people who do not accept consuming any kind of animal products including dairy products obviously I see your point. Modern farming practices are a major ethical problem. Ideally we would nourish ourselves in a way that causes as few problems as possible for other species, but I feel that whatever we do it will be a compromise. From hearing people's experiences over the years I have come to the conclusion that for most people, in order to sustain their nutrition long term, they need to supplement a plant based diet with fortified foods, various supplements, dairy products, eggs or even insects.

One way of bringing this nutrition in is by consumption of moderate amounts of raw dairy products such as milk, butter, cheese, yoghurt and kefir from as ethical a source as possible. The grazing animals convert the grasses, herbs and insects together with the sun energy they absorb from grazing naked outside into a form of nutrition that we can utilise, especially if it is fermented or cultured in the form of cheese, yoghurt or kefir. These days ethical dairy farms who do not take the young mammals from their mothers are beginning to appear and I suspect this will be a trend. The only thing stopping this is our willingness to pay the extra for the products that this requires.

Another issue to consider is whether the milk is A1 or A2 type. A2 is the heirloom milk from goats, sheep or Jersey, Guernsey, African or Asian cows and is way more suitable for human consumption than so-called A1 type milk. A1 milk is modern milk from Friesian or Holstein cows. It is different and mutated. One of the amino acids, proline, has been replaced with histidine which causes an allergic reactions in some people which can cause long term problems. This is actually one of the reasons so many people are 'allergic to dairy'. If you use raw A2 milk and ferment it, many people who considered themselves dairy intolerant are, in fact, not. They are just allergic to the altered biochemistry of the milk. Cooking or pasteurising milk makes it less digestible and coagulates the proteins. Fermenting the milk to make yoghurt or kefir (a powerful variation on live yoghurt), on the other hand, breaks down the casein and lactose and makes it more digestible. This is particularly helpful for people with lactose intolerance. Even people who traditionally struggle with dairy produce will often find that raw A2 type milk, cultured into kefir or yoghurt will work for them.

Eating fish or meat in any substantial way does present a problem in terms of steroid hormones. We are also not really designed to digest flesh foods. However some people report that they do not thrive without them. There may be specific substances in meat that can be taken in the form of supplements instead such as CoQ10. Traditional people ate animal products as sparingly and respectfully as possible and used all parts of the animal to avoid waste and unnecessary killing. This also provided more complete nutrition. Fish nowadays can be overloaded with toxic metals such as mercury too. That's a terrible shame for them and also a terrible shame for us if we eat them.

To succeed with a vegan diet the important nutrients to supplement with are the fat soluble vitamins which are generally not found in plant foods. These are vitamin D, which is essential for the metabolism of calcium, and K2 which is needed for vitamin D to do it's work. In temperate latitudes we cannot metabolise vitamin D from the sun in the winter months because the sun is not high enough to supply us with UVB wavelengths. Many people, especially females have difficulty converting the plant form of vitamin A (betacarotene) into retinol and this may need to be supplemented, though in moderation, as it is toxic in too large quantities. B12, iodine, iron for women and children , DHA and EPA are also essential. DHA and EPA are forms of omega 3 fatty acids that the neural system must have. In theory we should be able to convert them from the plant forms of omega 3 but in practice this does not happen sufficiently in most people.

Some people consider eggs an ethical option if they are laid unfertilised by truly free range hens. Eggs contain the nutritional factors that are missing from plant foods and if you like them I feel they can be very helpful, as long as they are good quality fresh, truly free range and organic. Raw egg whites block the absorption of the B vitamin biotin, but raw egg yolks can be added to smoothies and other dishes. There is another view that if you eat fertilised eggs this problem with the whites is avoided.

The issue of animal foods is an ongoing debate. I merely my job to point out the nutrition we need to thrive and rebuild our neural systems.

Commonalities of the Weston Price Diets

I feel this is a useful list to share and helps clarify what we need to remain nourished in all this food experimenting. It is taken from Weston Price. We are in a new situation today with the supplements we have available and the ability to ship goods around the world, so we can create new ways of covering these dietary commonalities.

The diets of healthy primitive and non-industrialised peoples contain no refined or denatured foods such as refined sugar or corn syrup; white flour; canned foods; pasteurised, homogenised, skimmed or low-fat milk; refined or hydrogenated vegetable oils; protein powders; artificial vitamins or toxic additives and colourings.

All traditional cultures consume some sort of animal protein and fat from fish and other seafood; water and land fowl; land animals; eggs; milk and milk products; reptiles; and insects.

Primitive diets contain at least four times the calcium and other minerals and ten times the fat soluble vitamins from animal fats (vitamin A, vitamin D and the Price Factor–now believed to be vitamin K2) as the average American diet.

In all traditional cultures, some animal products are eaten raw.

Primitive and traditional diets have a high food-enzyme content from raw dairy products, raw meat and fish; raw honey; tropical fruits; cold-pressed oils; wine and unpasteurised beer; and naturally preserved, lacto-fermented vegetables, fruits, beverages and condiments.

Seeds, grains and nuts are soaked, sprouted, fermented or naturally leavened in order to neutralise naturally occurring anti-nutrients in these foods, such as phytic acid, enzyme inhibitors, tannins and complex carbohydrates.Total fat content of traditional diets varies from 30% to 80% but only about 4% of calories come from polyunsaturated oils naturally occurring in grains, pulses, nuts, fish, animal fats and vegetables. The balance of fat calories is in the form of saturated and monounsaturated fatty acids.

Traditional diets contain nearly equal amounts of omega-6 and omega-3 essential fatty acids.

All primitive diets contain some salt.

Traditional cultures consume animal bones, usually in the form of gelatine rich bone broths.

Traditional cultures make provisions for the health of future s by providing special nutrient-rich foods for parents-to-be, pregnant women and growing children; by proper spacing of children; and by teaching the principles of right diet to the young.

Blood Types

I used to be skeptical about the concept of eating according to blood type introduced in 'Eat Right 4 Your Type' by Dr Peter D'Adamo and Catherine Whitney, until I saw how many people it helped and was relevant to. You can still apply the principles here whatever your blood type, adjusting them according to your needs. It's another factor to weave in. As with the Weston Price Information we can practice it in new ways with the options we have today. For example if you need a lot of protein it can be at least partially plant based.

Food Quality and Combining

Food combining is a question that often comes up. Basically if you imagine the digestive system as a long tube, we need to put faster digesting foods in before slower digesting ones. This means fruit before other foods as our bodies to digest it very quickly. A swiftly assimilated food such as melon should be eaten alone and before any other foods. So ideally, we would not include melon in a fruit salad. Mono-eating - eating several of one fruit with nothing else does have a feeling of lightness about it. Many foods can be combined well, for example blended seeds and fruits because seeds are part of fruit. The thing is just to be aware of this issue and see what works for you.

Obviously I recommend organic food where possible. This is more crucial with some foods than others i.e. the ones that are likely to be heavily sprayed. Strawberries, tomatoes and greens spring to mind. Carrots and cucumbers taste very different if they are organic. Bear in mind the country of origin too. It can take a little research, but certain crops in certain countries simply aren't chemically sprayed. Then there may be local producers who don't want to pay for organic certification but who are not spraying.

Freshness is nearly as important as not being heated above biological temperature. Of course in our original state food went straight from plant to mouth without spoilage.

I want to mention the alkaline issue here too. Our diet should ideally be predominantly though not all alkalising foods. This is a reference to the mineral content of the food. There are foods such as citrus fruit which are acidic but within the body are alkalising. Citrus fruit and greens are the most alkalising foods we generally eat. Grains, seeds and heavy protein foods tend to be acidifying. Adding citrus fruit and green leaves into recipes and meals can really help balance them and make us feel much better.

In the morning after we wake up the body is naturally in a cleansing cycle. There is a lot to be said for eating easily digestible foods such as fruit and smoothies for the first part of the day. It is possible to get in a lot of energy this way and keep a very clear head.

Recommended Food List

I recommend a diet composed of the following food groups for optimal health and brain nutrition. This list is designed to cover the amino acids (proteins), carbohydrates, fats, mineral and vitamins that we need plus other micronutrients.

Fruit - including tropical fruit such as bananas, mangoes, figs, papayas, and pineapple and durian - if you can obtain it. Melons, apricots, apples, pears, plums, cherries, kakis, grapes, currants, oranges, lemons, grapefruit. Non sweet fruit such as avocados, olives, tomatoes, cucumber. Berries such as strawberries, raspberries, blueberries, blackberries and so forth.

Nuts and Seeds – we do not digest the seeds in the fruit we eat nowadays plus the seeds of the fruits we eat are often under-formed and we tend to discard them. We can make up for this by eating the seeds of other foods. Seeds are easier to digest than nuts and nuts should be eaten in moderation but both nuts and seeds give us dense nutrition. They should generally be soaked in water for a few hours before use to break down their growth inhibitors which interfere in digestion and assimilation of nutrients. Hemp is the one seed that does not contain many growth inhibitors but soaking helps rehydrate the seed anyway. Include a wide variety. Hemp is a good staple, also eat sunflower seeds, pumpkin seeds, sesame seeds, hazels (filberts), walnuts, almonds, coconut., cedar or pine nuts, macadamias, Brazils and pecans.

Greens - needed for minerals, chlorophyll and protein and various co-factors, they also alkalise the body in a way that counteracts the acid-forming properties of most nuts and seeds and some other foods. Dark greens are particularly nutritious. If you have the time and inclination you can juice wild greens such as nettles in spring. Growing sprouts such as alfalfa, quinoa and radish is a cost effective way to get in highly vitalising vegetable matter too. For super busy people good quality dried green vegetable powders with grasses, hemp and other green leaves and algae are also a convenient way. Root vegetables such as carrots and sweet potatoes are very nutritious and grated help fill out a salad. A large salad with organic leaves is an important meal each day.

Sea vegetables – provide iodine and trace minerals which are more abundant in the oceans than the land. Kelp is the richest in iodine.

Oils – you get some but not all your fatty acids from nuts and seeds. It's important to keep a good balance between omega 3 and omega 6 essential fatty acids. Flaxseed (linseed) oil can help with this, or other omega supplements. By the way, cold pressed oils that have not gone rancid are generally pleasant to taste. Plant extracted omega 3 oils have to be converted inside us to provide EPA and DHA, omega fatty acids which the brain needs. Coconut oil can help this process. For most people the conversion process is not efficient enough though and you need to add in EPA (Eicosapentaenoic acid) and DHA (Docosahexaenoic acid) with purified fish oil or an algae supplement. These forms of omega are needed by the brain and this is why traditionally fish was said to be good for intelligence. To eat enough fish to get the EPA and DHA we need would overload the body in the toxins because of the heavy metals they now carry.

Raw Dairy Products or Equivalent Foods - I talked about the need for either moderate amounts of animal products or suitable supplements containing the nutrients that are difficult or impossible to obtain from plant sources. Raw goats and cows milk, goats' and cows' butter, sheep or goats' yoghurt, kefir, unpasteurised cheese, raw (and carefully selected organic, free-range) egg yolks all contain fat soluble vitamins.   In temperate latitudes, for much of the year, the sun does not rise high enough to give us the UVB light our skin needs to make sufficient vitamin D. B12 needs also to come from animal sources - plant sourced B12 is not the form humans need and can even get in the way of proper B12 absorption. The benefits of Vitamin A in the form of retinol include eyesight and skin. Most women in have difficulty converting the plant form betacarotene into retinol. Dairy products have had a diminished reputation over the years because of their quality and farming practices. In earlier centuries raw milk was recommended as a recuperating drink in a similar way green juice is today. If you think about it - grazing animals naked in the sunlight, consuming grasses, herbs and insects produce this amazing maternal liquid with the goodness of the greens plus insect material, that we as mammals potentially have the ability to digest. The loss of the sense of symbiotic connection between humans and animals and the farming and food production practices that have come about have changed things for sure, but I do want to make this point. There are many nutritional impacts on the milk and milk products. Pasteurisation takes food above biological temperature just as cooking does. When milk is pasteurised it is denatured, it simply is not the same food as raw milk. The proteins and fats are not digestible in the same way. Add to this the issue of A1 milk. The milk from modern cattle has a histidine molecule where there is a proline molecule in heirloom and goat's and sheep's milks. This can be allergenic and is part of what is behind modern milk's bad reputation. If you take A2 milk from Jersey or Guernsey cows or goats or sheep's milk, keep it raw and then ferment it you have a very different food that most people can digest and utilise. Kefir, I talk about later and is a stunning example of this.

Super high nutrient foods, Supplements and Tonic Herbs - due to poor quality of soil (including organic because of long term soil erosion), fruit being picked unripe, storage and the fact that the human gut is not working at its best, we need all the help we can get. Plus due to our anomalous fast ageing process our body slows down in making some essential substances for body function by our thirties and we can supplement to compensate for that. This is the case whether eating cooked or raw food. You can obtain extra minerals, vitamins and healthy mood enhancing compounds from superfoods and supplements. Food and herb sources are best where possible. The minerals we are most likely to be low on include sulphur, zinc, iron (for women and children), magnesium, silicon, selenium and iodine and we could do with much higher doses of vitamin C and the B vitamins than most people get. High nutrient foods with special properties such as rosehip, mesquite, algarroba, pollen, gojis, purple corn, noni, sea greens enhance diet although they cannot be a replacement for basic nutrition. MSM (natural sulphur) is worth taking as I described earlier. MSM naturally occurs in rainwater but, unless we grow most or our own food, this is lost in along the way in the journey our food makes to us. Aloe vera contains some invaluable elements such as monatomic elements; the fresh gel is ideal and the plants are easy to grow on a window sill. E3 Live is a great all round supplement, so nourishing that many people find it helps with weight loss. A high quality plant derived mineral supplement including the full range of trace minerals is also advisable.

Water - of course our main constituent - it is well known now that we should drink plenty of good water – I feel that clean fresh spring water is the ideal. It does not need to be drunk alone – it is an excellent carrier for other super-nutrition in the form of teas, elixirs, juices, smoothies etc.

Fermented foods provide probiotics and B vitamins and can be revolutionary in our health. Fermenting food also creates ATP, adenosine triphosphate, energy-carrying molecules which capture chemical energy obtained from the breakdown of food molecules and release it to fuel other cellular processes. Fermented foods include coconut and milk kefirs, cultured vegetables such as sauerkraut and kimchee, miso and seed cheeses.

Medicinal mushrooms – reishi and shitake have become well known. Also chaga, lion's mane, tremella etc all boost the immune system and have many other health enhancing qualities. They contain natural sugars called polysaccharides.

Flowers – many flowers are edible, they are the precursors of fruit. Nasturtium, borage flowers and rose petals are examples to use in salad.

Thirty very Magical Foods

We are so lucky to live in this Earthly paradise. Eating the foods that are freely gifted to us to nourish, heal and protect us, makes this real for us. It connects us with the land and its incredible wisdom. Forming relationships with these fruits, seeds, leaves, roots, pods, and cultures we see beyond food as inert building blocks and realise that they, like us, are intricate arrays of complex biochemical components. These interact with our own neurochemistry to affect our thoughts feelings and actions. We are, by nature, in relationship with plant and microorganisms There are so many magical foods and herbs, I could have gone on forever with this list but decided to stop at thirty. Enough to give a flavour. You can bring more of these foods into you life in the recipes later in the book.

Kefir

Kefir is an incredible magic food which comes into being through the symbiotic activities of three living groups: humans, grazing animals and beneficial micro-organisms. The name 'kefir' means 'good feeling', an apt name as it contains a lot of tryptophan from which serotonin, the well-being biochemical, is made. It's origins remain mysterious, outside the usual descriptions of how life forms came about, and this adds to it's allure. Stories of goats' udders rubbing on fungi in the fields, and that it is a gift from the divine are explanations I have come across. The kefir culture itself, needs both the animals and humans to continue its' life journey.

Milk kefir and water kefir are two different kinds of SCOBY (symbiotic culture of yeast and bacteria). Milk kefir needs to be fed a raw animal milk on a long term basis in order to thrive, whilst water kefir needs a sugar solution such as sugar water, fruit juice or coconut water. Here I first describe milk kefir.

Kefir can be thought of as a kind of powerful yoghurt but with some significant advantages. It is the most powerfully probiotic food or supplement that we know of. It actively repopulates the gut, laying down a healthy mucus layer that micro-flora can flourish in, supporting the digestive and immune system. Yoghurt contains transient bacteria that keep the digestive system clean and provide food for the friendly bacteria that reside there. But kefir can actually colonise the intestinal tract. This makes it a valuable help in the case of candida.

The culture is so powerful that, unlike yoghurt, it can successfully compete with all the micro-organisms that naturally exist in milk and also it will work at room temperature. This means that, unlike with yoghurt, the milk does not have to be heated to make it and so the nutritional components in the milk remain undamaged. This is great because it allows us to take full advantage of the nutrition in dairy milk, for example the fat soluble vitamins A (retinol), D3 and K2. Also it avoids the changes to the proteins and sugars in milk which can cause problems.

The kefir culture, which transforms animal milks into a supremely nourishing drink, is actually a mixture of numerous kinds of friendly bacteria and yeasts. Our bodies are really whole ecosystems and ideally our digestive tracts contain ten times more friendly micro-organisms than we have cells in our bodies; these support a healthy immune system and brain function. The kefir culture itself is potentially immortal – if properly looked after and fed with milk, it can live indefinitely. The liquid kefir that it makes is a preserved living food and can keep for months. We prefer to store it in a cool place but this is not necessary. If it is stored in a warm place secondary fermentation in the bottle will take place so you may want to check that too much pressure is not building up over time.

The particular nutritive properties of kefir are numerous. The culture rebalances the amino acids in animal milk making them more suitable for humans. In particular, as already mentioned, it increases the amount of tryptophan which is the raw material from which serotonin is made. Tryptophan tends to be lacking in modern diets as it is easily damaged by cooking. Kefir contains ample amounts of B vitamins including B12. Acetylcholine in it improves sleep and is good for memory, intelligence, learning, enthusiasm and general mood. Kefir also contains lecithin which helps in the assimilation of fats. It contains 'right-rotating' lactic acid (as opposed to 'left-rotating' lactic acid found in other yoghurts) which revives cells.

One of the great aspects of kefir is that it allows us to take advantage of the nutrition in raw milk whilst avoiding some of the potential allergenic problems of dairy products. The culture breaks down the lactose into lactic acid and the casein into beneficial peptides. Kefir is best made with Jersey or Guernsey, goats milk or other traditional A2 type heirloom milks.. Drinking kefir consistently for a few weeks has been known to clear up residual dairy intolerance. Note that kefir is a powerful healing agent and it is wise to begin with very small amounts, say a tablespoon, building up to about half a pint a day. As the body readjusts it's ecology and throws out unwanted materials there can be a mild healing reaction. Milk from animals that are grass fed for most of the year is especially nutritious and of course this is a kinder way to treat the animals.. It is also interesting to note that kefir can break down pesticides.

Added to all this, kefir has an unusual, delicious and acquired taste. When bottled, as this product is, it undergoes a secondary fermentation and becomes slightly fizzy - the 'champagne of raw dairy'.

Kefir scobies, the so-called 'grains' are living things; they are potentially immortal if cared for and fed properly and can be used indefinitely. They continue to grow (doubling in size about every 16 days) and the extra culture can given away or even eaten. Milk kefir can be made with coconut milk, but the scoby itself needs raw animal milks in order to flourish and grow, so it is wise to feed the grains animal milk by making a batch in this way regularly, even if you yourself want to drink coconut kefir. We come back to the methodology of making kefir in the Recipes chapter.

Water kefir culture is sometimes called Tibiscos. It is a different Scoby. It is a great alternative for those who do not wish to drink milk kefir as it is also a probiotic. It needs to be fed liquids containing sugar such as sugar water, fruit juice, or coconut water. Some people use fructose water of fruit blended with water. Coconut juice/water is our favourite. It's simple and clean. You can purchase both kinds of cultures in many places nowadays including online.

Hemp and CBD

Hemp is an amazing plant with a unique role to play in human nutrition. The seeds, leaves and CBD oils, which are extracted from the whole plant all have astonishing benefits. People often ask what is the difference between hemp and cannabis. Simply put they are the same species. Hemp is the old northern European name for the cannabis plant and now the word is used to denote strains of cannabis that are low in THC (tetrahydrocannabinol) and hence legal to grow in many places, at least with a license. Its history is interesting. In Elizabethan England, landowners were under a legal obligation to grow it because of it's importance for materials used by the navy. Hemp converts the sun's energy into cellulose through photosynthesis faster than any other plant. Recently the benefits of hemp CBD oil, for helping with many health situations have become widely known. The oil from the seeds, the seeds themselves and the leaves also have great nutritional properties.

Hemp leaf is exceptionally alkalising at the cellular level and is an extraordinarily complex superfood, containing many of the essential nutrients in good ratios. It is rich in minerals, essential natural sugars (glyconutrients), chlorophyll and silicon. It brings light energy into the body and energises the brain. It provides, amongst other nutrients, essential natural sugars and carbohydrates, invaluable to sports people. It also helps with melanin production in the skin and helps one absorb full spectrum light. It is low in THC (tetrahydrocannabinol). However it is still rich in other helpful cannabinoids, in particular CBD (cannabidiol).

Dried hemp leaf powder is, unlike most green superfoods, delicious blended into smoothies and raw chocolates, even enhancing the taste.

Hemp seeds, especially made into hemp milk (see recipes section) provide a comprehensive array of amino acid and fatty acids, with a good ratio of omega 3 to omega 6. You can also obtain these fatty acids form cold pressed hemp oil, not to be confused with CBD oil or cannabis oil.

CBD oil is a term for a vegetable oil, for example olive oil or avocado oil which has been infused with the hemp plant, using a process which extracts the cannabinoids from the hemp plant into the oil. This is the medicinal oil.

CBD stands for cannabidiol. In fact cannabidiol belongs to a whole category of over 80 compounds called cannabinoids found in the cannabis sativa or hemp plant. CBD has become well known in recent times for its remarkable healing properties. Cannabinoids are very similar to a group of chemicals in the human body which regulate the way the body runs and remains healthy. For historical reasons these endogenous (originating within) compounds have been named endo-cannabinoids. The reason is that they were studied in the cannabis plant before they were identified in the human body. Cannabinoids from the hemp plant latch onto the same receptors sites as the endo-cannabinoids produced in the human body, so create a similar effect and help regulate the bodily systems in a very beneficial way.

As described in this book, over millennia humans have moved away from their natural lifestyle and diet and connection with the healing power of the Earth, As a result we have developed deficiencies and glitches in the way our bodies work which have been passed on epigenetically through the generations. Healing plants contain compounds that can help this situation, none more so than hemp with its ability to reactivate the human endocannabinoid system.

Also, addressing a specific modern problem, the high quantities of THC in highly bred strains of cannabis often used nowadays, can bring on anxiety and paranoia. The original plant (to which all cannabis and hemp will tend if allowed to seed and regrow naturally) is well-balanced with the anti-psychotic cannabinoid, CBD. Hemp leaf is low in THC but has plenty of CBD so can be a very healing medicine food.

Figs

Figs are one of the most popular foods amongst primates including humans in areas where they grow. They contain ample amounts of a very important class of biochemicals called mono-amine oxidase inhibitors (MAOI's) which have a very significant impact on our state of mind. Mono-amine oxidase (MAO) is an enzyme which breaks down the monoamine neurotransmitters in our brains which include serotonin, dopamine etc. Mono-amine oxidase inhibitors slow the break down and so boost the levels of these neurotransmitters.

Added to this, at least one of the mono-amine neurotransmitters, norepinephrine, stimulates the pineal gland. This causes the pineal gland to produce more of its hormones. These hormones have a pivotal effect on human development and our states of mind. It is possible that the presence of the powerfully influential chemicals in figs may be the underlying reason why the fig tree had significance to the ancient mystics.

Figs are one of the oldest cultivated plants, having been grown since at least 5000BC. The symbiotic relationship between humans and fruit trees is one we still sense to day.

Figs are one of the most densely mineralised of all fruits, being particularly high in calcium, also potassium, magnesium and iron. In the wild they contain a lot of insect material which is highly nutritious.

Noni

Noni, a cherished fruit of the South Pacific, has been used for natural healing for generations. It has a reputation for helping with all kinds of ailments and addictions, promoting general good health, high levels of energy and well-being. It is said to boost the immune system and cell health, cleanse the body of harmful bacteria and purify the blood.

One of noni's active constituents is pro-xeronine which the body makes into xeronine. Xeronine is an important nutrient which tends to be lacking in the modern diet. By consuming noni we can redress this situation. One of xeronine's functions is to allow better absorption of amino acids such as tryptophan which makes serotonin in the brain. So how does noni help with addictions? In many plants xeronine is stored for its nitrogen, clumped together with 'molecular garbage'. The compounds formed are part of a class of compounds called alkaloids. Over 10,000 alkaloids are known to exist in various plants. These include nicotine, caffeine, cocaine, heroin and morphine. These alkaloids are completely inactive in the plant but because they resemble xeronine they are treated and accepted as xeronine by the proteins in our bodies. However our bodies adapt to these alkaloids by slightly changing the shape of the proteins so they will fit with the alkaloid being used rather than xeronine. Thus we become dependent on the alkaloid in question i.e. addicted. By using noni you can flood your body with xeronine. By doing this you make yourself less likely to crave the alkaloids mentioned.

Coconut Oil

Coconut is one of the oldest and most popular foods known. It contains the valuable healthy saturated fats that are so nourishing and essential for our brains and nervous systems. It has been eaten by humans for a long long time. Coconut oil is liquid at tropical temperature and sets in temperate climates, where it is sometimes known as coconut butter, not to be confused with creamed coconut. Coconut fat contains raw medium chain fatty acids that the body efficiently converts to energy rather than storing as fat. It's a great body and brain fuel, especially for those who struggle with sugars. This is one reason it is of such benefit for seniors' brain function. It also boosts the metabolism by supporting the thyroid, thus helping with weight loss. It improves insulin secretion and balances sugar levels in the blood. It's a nutritional precursor to the anti-ageing hormone pregnenolene. It improves digestion and absorption of nutrients.

Coconut oil also cleanses. It cleans out toxic fats deposits. It can help the body utilise essential fatty acids e.g. omega 3's, omega 6's and phospholipids such as choline and lecithin. It is anti-oxidant, antiviral, anti-fungal, antimicrobial, and helps kill parasites. Used for oil pulling it draws out bacteria and so helps protect teeth and gums. Swirl a large chunk around your mouth for about twenty minutes in the morning, spit it out and rinse with clean water.

You can apply it externally on the skin too. It makes skin look wonderful and also helps heal sunburn, along with aloe.

Cacao

Known as ';Food of the Gods', traditionally cacao or cocoa was consumed as a cooked chocolate drink, including ingredients such as corn (maize) and chilli. It's origins are in Mexico, in the 'chocolate belt', the latitudes close enough to the equator for the cocoa trees to grow. Since then the cocoa trees have been hybridised but it still possible to obtain heirloom varieties. There are actually three different types of cacao used in chocolate production today. Two hundred years ago criollo was the predominant cacao bean; it has become scarcer now as it is less resistant to disease so now the more robust Forastero dominates the world-wide market. The Trinitario is a hybrid between Criollo and Forastero, developed in Trinidad to survive the conditions there and now used to produce most fine flavour cocoa. More rare to find today, it was a Criollo that was the original fine flavour cacao. It has a particular reddish tinge and a complex taste, including hints of nuts, caramel and vanilla.

There is some wonderful biochemistry in cacao that may be more active when it is not heat treated. There are also arguments for heating to break down compounds in chocolate that may be problematic in large quantities. In any case it's wise not to become a chocolate addict, as the Aztecs were reputed to be, abut rather enjoy it as a treat. I have noticed that some people, especially women, can become hooked into it as their main source of magnesium. If you get plenty of magnesium from other foods, or supplementing then you relationship with chocolate can remain fun. One of the great advantages of the wave of raw chocolate that came in a few years back is that it was made with sweeteners that are not sugar. Now sugar is creeping back in. Maybe not standard white sugar, but sugars nonetheless. Lucuma, honey or maple syrup are sweeteners I would recommend as wholefoods that have health benefits. Raw chocolate is easy to make when you know how and there are recipes at the end of this book.

Raw cacao contains many active biochemicals which combine to produce the lovely feelings described by many as similar to those of being in love. Phenylethylamine (PEA) creates feelings of, excitement and euphoria. It is abundant in the brain when we are happy, aroused, interested in something that really captivates our attention or generally in love with life. Dopamine levels also increase in response to DEA. Dopamine is the biochemical messenger of motivation, enthusiasm and desire for life's experiences. Anandamide, known as the 'bliss chemical' because it makes us feel so good is also present in raw cacao, along with breakdown inhibitors which prolong its circulation in the brain. Monoamine oxidase inhibitors which keep our neurotransmitter levels high are also abundant. The biochemistry in raw cacao also includes lots of antioxidants and large amounts of magnesium, a very important mineral for the heart and muscle flexibility. In terms of brain biochemistry, raw cacao contains ample amounts of the essential amino acid tryptophan which works with magnesium and vitamins B6 and B3 to produce serotonin, the neurotransmitter associated with pleasure and feeling good. Tryptophan is easily damaged by heating so this is an effect experienced more with raw cacao than standard chocolate.

Sunflower Seeds

It's at least partly the ability of the sunflower to turn to face the sun and absorb so much of its energy that gives them such a high nutritional value. They are particularly high in B and E vitamins and the minerals iron, zinc and calcium, also choline. Choline is a chemical precursor or building block needed to produce the neurotransmitter acetylcholine, important for memory, intelligence and mood. The vitamin D synthesised from the sunshine helps in the utilisation of the calcium. Sunflower seeds are also high in fatty acids such as linoleic acid and amino acids (protein). Together with the B vitamins these boost the adrenal glands and so sunflower seeds are an ideal snack in times of an energy slump or stress. Sunflower seeds are useful for overcoming a smoking habit because nicotine also boosts the level of adrenal hormones. Eating a handful or two when the smoking urge kicks in mimics the effect of the nicotine. Like nicotine, sunflower seeds, with their B vitamins and various sedative oils, have a soothing effect on the nervous system. Like nicotine, sunflower seeds trigger the release of glycogen from the liver, producing a lift in brain activity and mood.

Sunflower seeds nourish the digestive system and pancreas and contain a high concentration of lipotropic or fat moving constituents, so assist the liver in metabolising fats and removing them from the bloodstream. Used in combination with sesame seeds and pumpkin seeds, sunflower seeds provide a particularly good balance of essential amino acids.

Sunflowers are native to Peru and Mexico. Sunflower was a common crop among Native American tribes going back to at least 3000 BC and they used the seeds in breads. In Peru the flowers were much revered by the Aztecs. In the Aztec temples of the Sun, the priestesses were crowned with sunflowers and carried them in their hands. Spanish explorers took the sunflower plant to Europe in the 1500's, where it was widely used as an ornamental plant. It was in Russia that it was rediscovered as food plant in the early 19th century. Sunflowers can be used to extract toxic ingredients such as lead, arsenic, uranium and caesium-137 and strontium-90 from soil and water and were used after the Chernobyl disaster.

The florets within the sunflower's cluster are arranged in a spiral pattern, whereby each floret is oriented toward the next by approximately the golden angle, This pattern produces the most efficient packing of seeds within the flower head. The sunflower seeds collected and sold for planting are actually the fruit of the plant. The inedible husk is the wall of the fruit and the true seed lies within the kernel. The sunflower seeds sold for human consumption are the kernels.

Seeds should ideally be soaked for a few hours and drained before eating to remove enzyme inhibitors. Sunflower seeds are delicious left an extra day to sprout and can also be grown into sunflower greens in a layer of soil in the kitchen. They can be added to smoothies to make them rich and creamy. They also are great in dehydrated raw burgers, breads and seed cheeses.

Pumpkin Seeds

Pumpkin seeds are one of the most concentrated plant food sources of zinc. Zinc is crucial role for growth and cell division and many body functions. It is one of the most likely minerals for us to be deficient in because it is quite difficult for the body to absorb and it is particularly depleted in overworked soils.

Zinc is important in hormone production, the male prostate gland and sperm production. It improves the sense of taste and smell and is good for the skin, immune system, muscles, appetite regulation, memory, energy and mental clarity.

Raw pumpkin seeds are also one of the best natural sources of tryptophan which tends to be deficient in people's diets because it is destroyed by cooking. Zinc is involved in the processing of serotonin from tryptophan, so pumpkin seeds help improve mood.

Pumpkin seeds contain an amino acid cucurbitin which lessen the damage sometimes caused by testosterone to the prostate gland and male hair growth. The same amino acid rids the body of parasites by loosening their grip. Pumpkin seeds are helpful with bladder problems because they contain a phytochemical (natural plant compound) called curbita which calms the bladder and acts as a diuretic.

As well as zinc they are also rich in iron, calcium and magnesium, other key minerals that are often deficient. Of course the amount of these minerals in the seeds will depend on the concentration of minerals in the soil in which the pumpkins grow. Pumpkin seeds contain B vitamins, particularly B17, with its reputed ability to prevent tumours. The fatty acids in the seeds, particularly omega 3's improve the quality of skin and protect it from damage from UV radiation.

Interestingly, pumpkin seeds inhibit the effects of aromatase, lessening the damaging impact of testosterone on the brain described earlier and also helping control oestrogen levels.

The pumpkin seeds generally available from health-food shops are from shell-less, dark green varieties. Like other seeds they are best soaked for a few hours before eating to remove growth inhibitors

Berries

Strawberries, raspberries, blackberries and blueberries, feel such natural foods to be eating and they are. In a world of hybridised and over sweet fruits them are gems. It's so wonderful to find blackberries or tiny flavoursome wild strawberries growing in the countryside. Fortunately now we can eat them all year. It's fine to use frozen berries too. In fact these may sometimes be the freshest ones available at certain times of year. Berries contain vitamins including C and many other phytochemicals. A few are particularly worth mentioning. Nearly all berry seeds, blackberry, elderberry, raspberry, cranberry and strawberry contain B17 and if you finely blend them in smoothies this is released. B17 is a controversial nutrient which I come back to a little later.

Blueberries

Moving onto some more specific berries, blueberries stand out for their exceptional ability to stimulate brain tissue growth, known as neurogenesis. Blueberries contain polyphenols, especially the blue flavonoids anthocyanins, also found in blackberries and black currants.
"The four most outstanding foods for stimulating neurogenesis [brain growth] are blueberries, omega-3 fatty acids, green tea and curcumin...It's hard to sing blueberries' praises highly enough. Blueberries act in so many ways to promote neurogenesis and protect the brain from cognitive decline that if blueberries were a drug, pharmaceutical companies would be bombarding us with ads to entice us to upgrade our brain with this 'miracle drug'...blueberries seem to protect against cognitive decline, inflammation, oxidation (free radical damage), radiation, and glycation. Generally it takes different substances to protect against any one of these things. That blueberries have so many effects is little short of astounding...blueberries allow better communication among neurons, something called signal transduction, and they protect against brain injury, stroke, certain neurotoxins, excitotoxicity" says Brant Cortwight in his highly useful book 'Neurogenesis'.

Strawberries

Strawberries are so well loved and their health benefits match, including improved eye care, proper brain function, relief from high blood pressure, arthritis, gout and various cardiovascular diseases. The impressive polyphenolic and antioxidant content of strawberries make them good for improving the immune system, preventing against various types of cancers, and for reducing the signs of premature ageing. They contain ample amounts of vitamin C and of course B17 in the seeds. They help to normalise blood sugar levels.

Strawberries are often thought of as a European fruit. They were used back in Roman times, and were first cultivated as a garden fruit in France in the 18th Century. However, they were also present in South American cultures much earlier.

Cherries

Cherries have been enjoyed for centuries and were eaten in ancient Rome, Greece, and China. It's thought that sweet cherries originated in Asia and were likely carried to Europe by birds. They are rich in antioxidants and are anti-inflammatory. They contain melatonin. Montmorency cherries are particularly rich in this, enough to be noticeable in effects.

Aloe

Much is written about the power of aloe online and elsewhere. When eaten raw it contains the monatomic elements rhodium and iridium, and also its incredible power to maintain youthful elastic skin and heal scars, lines and wrinkles. Applied after the sun it can prevent sunburn occurring and its capacity to heal wounded skin never ceases to amaze me. You can apply externally and also eat a pea size amount - blended into smoothies if you like.

Vanilla

Vanilla has a relaxing effect. Stress causes inflammation, which releases inflammatory cytokines like TNF-alpha, which decreases your brain function. This is one of the reasons people don't perform well when they're stressed. Vanilla contains chemicals called vanilloids that activate receptors in a similar way to capsaicin in chillies. Thus vanilla is a cognitive enhancing agent.

Tomatoes

Although we now associate tomatoes with Italian cuisine, the tomato actually originated as a wild fruit 1300 years ago in the Aztec civilization of Ancient Mexico, known as tomatl in the Nahuatl language. It was central to the Aztecs' incredibly nutritious diet and alleged to give divine powers through the seeds. It was Spanish coloniser Hernán Cortés who conquered Tenochtitlan (present-day Mexico City) in 1521 and brought tomatoes to Europe. These early cultivated tomatoes were yellow and cherry-sized in form, and were called pommes d'or, pomi d'oro and goldapfel ("golden apples") in France, Italy and Germany respectively. They have outstanding antioxidant content and high concentration of lycopene which is excellent for bone health. They are great for the immune system and contain vitamins A (betacarotene), C, and K, as well as significant amounts of vitamin B6, folate, and thiamin. Tomatoes are also a good source of potassium, manganese, magnesium, phosphorous, and copper.

Cucumbers

Cucumbers are hydrating and a great source of silicon, a beauty mineral, which makes our hair thick, our nails strong, and strengthens connective tissues and bones to improve flexibility. Silicon can improve the appearance of wrinkles, and can also increase the resilience of your skin. Be sure to buy organic cucumbers, because conventional cucumbers have a waxy coating on them to make them more visually appealing.

Lemons and Limes

Citrus fruits such as lemons, limes, oranges and grapefruit, while being in themselves acidic, alkalise the body with their minerals so counteract acid forming foods such as seeds and grains and make us feel great especially after exercise. Their acidic flavour rounds out the tastes of recipes. Limes add a tropical feel. They are rich in vitamin C and folate. Limonene, in the peel of lemons and limes, is amazing for metabolism, fat cleansing, improving digestion and is also calming.

Nettles

Nettles deserve a mention due to their extreme nutritional benefits and availability in so many places. I recommend juicing them. They make a great juice because they are extremely nutritious, are abundant, free, and mood lifting. You can combine with carrots, celery, cucumber and so forth, even adding ginger, lime and apple. Rich in minerals, alkalising, they boost the metabolism and serotonin levels and cleanse mucus. If you grasp them under the leaves they don't sting and certainly once you have juiced them their stings are gone! Use nettles in spring before they flower because the composition changes at this time. Pick just the very top of the nettle. It's worth picking a couple of large bags of them as a small amount of concentrated juice is produced.

Chlorella and Spirulina

Containing most of the nutrients that the body needs they are an ideal combination for renutrifying ourselves. They are especially useful in winter in Britain and Northern Europe when there are not so many wild greens around and also when traveling. They work to their maximum benefit if taken together. The suggested ratio is about two parts spirulina to one part of chlorella. Chlorella and spirulina are both algae, which are some of the earliest and simplest life forms on Earth. Because they are at the beginning of the food chain they accumulate far fewer toxins than other foods further up and, more than this, the large percentage of chlorophyll in both foods helps remove heavy metals and other toxins from the body.

Spirulina contains 67 – 71% protein, which is the highest of any food discovered including 18 amino acids and all 8 essential amino acid. The protein in spirulina is four times more absorbable than the protein in meat. Chlorophyll in spirulina helps remove heavy metals such as aluminium, cadmium, lead, arsenic, mercury and radioactive metals from the body. Containing ample calcium and magnesium, it has an alkalising effect on the body which protects the bones from the loss of alkalising minerals and also massively improves metabolic function. After human breast milk it is the no 1 food source of gamma-linolenic acid (GLA) which is necessary for a healthy nervous system. It's a blood builder containing chlorophyll and iron which together contain all the components of human blood. A powerful antioxidant, it also helps with blood sugar regulation because of its ideal ratio of protein, carbohydrates and fatty acids, which also helps curb cravings. It contains nucleic acids in RNA/DNA content enhance cellular renewal, growth and repair , vitamins A (beta-carotene), B1, B2, B6, E and K , phycocyanin, which is rare in other foods, enhances production of stem cells and so boosts the immune system and enhances the function of the brain and nervous system. The recommended dose for nutritional maintenance 10g a day; take up to 60g to fight disease or boost athletic performance

Chlorella contains 58% protein including all 8 essential amino acids. It contains more chlorophyll, at 3-5% than any other plant and so is a great detoxifier of heavy metals including mercury and radioactive elements. It also helps build blood. It's alkalising effect on the body protects the bones from the loss of alkalising minerals and also massively improves metabolic function. Polysaccharides in the cell wall bind with toxins such as pesticides and carry them safely out of body. They also stimulate interferon and anti-tumour activity. Chlorella growth factor (CGF) massively which boosts cell growth and the immune system and helps repair nerve tissues, increases the rate of rebuilding of tissues, boosts the immune system and restores the population of white blood cells, multiplies the growth of beneficial bacteria in the gut, and rebuilds nerve tissue and the liver. It contains vitamins C, E, B vitamins, folic acid and beta-carotene; it's extraordinarily rich in iron and calcium, and also contains iodine, magnesium and zinc. It is the highest known food source of RNA at 10% helping with regeneration and reducing ageing. The recommended dose: for nutritional maintenance 5g a day or more if it feels good.

Shilajit

Shilajit is a fascinating food substance, a dark brown mineral rich tar like substance that oozes out of rocks that have cracked due to the expansion and contraction of extreme weather conditions in the mountainous regions of Tibet, Nepal, China, Russia, Bhutan and Kashmir. There are different theories as to what shilajit is made of. One story goes that it is composed of humus and organic plant materials that have been compressed by layers of rock over millions of years from the time when the land where the Himalayas are now was a lush fertile garden valley. Another theory states that shilajit is the residue of plants, high in resin and latex, which had been degraded by bacteria or fungus. Yet another theory states it is the end result of rocks and soil broken down by mosses and liverworts.

It is sometimes sold as a paste and other times powdered for ease of use. It's an adaptogenic substance that can come in very handy as a tool against the stresses of a modern lifestyle. Plus it's incredibly rich in minerals laid down before the world pollution of modern times., just a lentil size amount in a day is enough. It adds a unique rich earthy flavour to chocolate elixirs.

Benefits include increasing bone density, building muscle mass, having better metabolism and brain function, a reduction in stiffness and calcification of the joints. It helps stabilise blood sugar, is anti-inflammatory, anti-ageing, and strengthens the immune system. Finally Shilajit is a potentiator, meaning it amplifies the ramps-up the beneficial effects and enhances their bio-availability and action of any substance it is used with.

Bee Pollen

Bee pollen is one of the oldest foods on the planet. It contains nearly all the nutrients that we are known to need and so theoretically we could live on just pollen and water. It also contains some beneficial and, as yet, unidentifiable substances. Studies have shown that consumption of bee products is common amongst long-lived people. It's a great energy food especially when you are busy. It has 25% protein including all 22 amino acids in highly bioavailable form making it one of the richest protein foods in nature. It contains all the vitamins except B12 and vitamins C, D, E and K. It has 28 – 60 minerals including some rare and valuable trace minerals depending on the flower pollen being used and a wide variety of fatty acids. It's rich in nucleic acids such as RNA and DNA which regenerate our cells. 15% lecithin which helps us assimilate fat and also contains phosphatidyl choline which is beneficial for the brain especially in growing children. It's a source of phenylalanine which regulates the appetite and balances metabolism so can help with weight loss., also rutin which helps strengthen blood vessels including capillaries with multiple health implications. It's the most enzyme rich product known on earth with strong antioxidant powers and is a natural antibiotic. It reduces the amount of histamine produced in response to an allergen.

Some people are actually allergic to bee pollen so try just a small amount the first time and build up slowly.

Goji Berries

Sometimes known as wolfberries, goji berries have been highly prized in China for over 2000 years as a longevity food. They are one of the most nutritious berries known. Gojis are the only food known to actually boost levels of human growth hormone (HGH) which then stimulates the production of other hormones, producing an overall rejuvenating and anti-ageing effect. They are an adaptogen, supporting the immune system and adrenal glands. Goji berries can be eaten as a snack food as you would raisins, or they can be blended into smoothies, soaked to make soups and savoury sauces and added to herbal teas for a delicious sweetness.

Nutrients found in goji berries include: complete protein including 19 amino acids, all 8 essential amino acids including the crucial phenylalanine and tryptophan (precursor of serotonin), over 21 minerals including zinc, which is so often deficient in our diets, iron and copper, antioxidants, particularly astaxanthin and lutein which protect and repair eyes

Lucuma

Lucuma is a delicious sweet caramel tasting sub-tropical fruit from Peru, similar to sapote. It is known as "the Gold of the Incas". The only reason we don't see the fresh fruit here is that it is not allowed to be exported from South America. In Peru lucuma is the favourite flavour of ice-cream and with good reason! Outside of South America we can use it as a dried powder, a delicious sweetener in drinks, smoothies, chocolate and desserts. It can be added to so many raw recipes much as you would add sugar to a cooked recipe, yet it is a healthy fruit. Nutritionally it contains: carbohydrates, vitamins - notably beta-carotene and niacin and minerals including iron.

Mediterranean Carob

Traditionally known as St John's Bread, carob is an incredibly mineral rich and sun-filled legume, growing in Mediterranean countries. It is abundant in lignans, a helpful kind of phytoestrogens found in fibre rich food. Raw carob is incredibly sweet and delicious. Helpful properties of carob include: it is rich in magnesium, calcium, potassium, iron, manganese, chromium, copper and selenium, 8% protein, vitamins A, B1, B2 and B3, pectin which absorbs toxins from the body and has a high fibre content for internal cleanliness. It contains lectins which are antiviral, anti-fungal, antibacterial and anti-inflammatory and it also balance hormones.
Sun-dried and powdered it's a great flavoursome substitute for people who find cacao too stimulating. It can also be mixed with cacao to enhance the flavour.

Yacon

Yacon is a South American relative of the sunflower with edible tubers and leaves. It is the tubers that are generally used, sliced, powdered or made into a syrup which tastes like malt syrup (but not necessarily raw). It's very delicious (more so than stevia and also malt syrup most would say) and sweet but the sweetness comes form fructose-oligosaccharides rather than sugars so it does not increase blood sugar levels very much, in other words it is a low-glycemic sweetener. It is also prebiotic meaning that it feeds friendly bacteria in the gut, including bifido-bacterium; so it helps the absorption of B vitamins and calcium. It is also antioxidant, rich in potassium and iron and strengthens the immune system.

Maca

Maca is a root that looks a little like a turnip. It grows in the mountains of Peru in highly variable conditions, including a wide temperature range, intense sunlight and high winds. It is know as an energy booster and an adaptogen, i.e. it helps the body deal with various stresses and also balances the body's nervous system, cardiovascular system and musculature. It is particularly known as a hormone balancer for both women and men. People often notice it's effects on their energy but it's wise to start with a small amount as it can also stimulate a detox.

Maca has been used by the inhabitants of Peru for thousands of years to enable them to deal with the challenging environment there. In recent years it has become popular further afield as a raw superfood. It goes well with cacao. It is an emulsifier and helps blend fats and waters smoothly, and so is a great flavour enhancer in drinks and elixirs and useful ingredient in raw recipes.

What are its properties in more detail? Well, it increases strength, stamina, energy and endurance. It increases neurotransmitter production and libido, supports the thyroid, contains the valuable fatty acids linolenic acid and oleic acid and is 10% protein including 18 amino acids and 7 essential amino acids. It is mineral rich including calcium, magnesium, phosphorous, potassium, sulphur, iron, zinc, iodine, copper and selenium. It contains vitamins B1 and B2.

As a cruciferous vegetable it provides detoxifying phytonutrients and it has some benefits in its raw form but like other cruciferous vegetables is best not eaten in large quantities raw every day. In Peru, its home, it is generally eaten cooked. You can buy gelatinised raw maca which is easier to digest because some of the starch is removed.

Psyllium

Psyllium husks are a wonderful ingredient for thickening raw sauces. The mucilage in them absorbs water. They have a benefit for cleansing too. When eaten they swell, absorbing toxins and easily carrying them out of the body. They can be used in combination with various herbal digestive cleanses.

Reishi and other Medicinal Mushrooms

Reishi mushrooms grow naturally in the wild, on live trees and decaying logs, in dense damp mountain woodlands. Known as the 'plant of immortality', in oriental medicine, reishi has been highly prized for its health properties. Now that ways have been found to cultivate them, reishi has become available to the masses. It boosts the immune system and is therefore a beneficial defence against all major disease. It is also calming - helping with sleep and keeping the mind and memory sharp. It can easily be incorporated into meals, added to soups and elixirs, sprinkled on salads and so forth. It is mentioned specifically in some of the recipes later on. Reishi is one of a large range of so called medicinal mushrooms. It's the mushroom mycelium powders that are generally used as they are more potent than the fruiting bodies. They include shitake, chaga, poria, himematsutake, cordyceps, lion's mane (which regenerates neural tissue), tremella (traditionally used by Chinese women for beautiful skin and possibly the most delicious medicinal mushroom). They all have their own individual properties and together work synergistically.

Stimulating your immune system with foods such as reishi and the other medicinal mushrooms is crucial too. These mushroom mycelia contain polysaccharides, natural sugars which feed the immune system. Disaccharide sugars such as cane sugar disable the immune system because they are similar in structure to vitamin C and compete for space with vitamin C which the white blood cells needs to destroy bacteria and viruses. This comes from the research by Linus Pauling in the 1970s to find out how the body uses Vitamin C. On the other hand the polysaccharides, beta glucans, found in foods such as medicinal mushrooms, bind and help specific immune cells to achieve a well-coordinated attack on their targets.

Black Turtle Beans

Beans such as black turtle beans are an example of beneficial cooked foods and are beans prized in Central and South America. The indigestible part of these beans feed beneficial bacteria in the colon which produce butyric acid. Cells lining the inside of the colon can use this butyric acid to fuel their many activities and keep the lower digestive tract functioning. Black beans are simple to prepare, you just cook in water for about an hour and they go well with tomatoes, peppers, onions , spices and other ingredients to make delicious meals.

Amazing Supplements for Health

Where do we draw the line between a food and a supplement? Of course in an unspoiled paradisiacal planet we would need no supplements. This is not now the case as we know. We need extras to provide what does not come from impoverished soils, what we miss out on from not living in our biological habitat, and the changes that come with our anomalous situation, whereby our bodies have stopped producing essential substances or stop producing them as we age in an unnaturally accelerated way. In this section I include supplements that you would definitely not think of as foods.

Zeolite Crystals and Iodine

I talk about these together simply because of their combined role in dealing with the worldwide radioactive toxicity of modern times that has come about after nuclear accidents and experimenting, toxic waste and wars. The impact is huge and we can protect ourselves in many ways. Here I highlight a few. Zeolite has come as a wonderful gift to us in these times of seemingly all-pervading pollution. Simply put, it is a volcanic rock that has been broken down into a fine powder so that is can pass into and out of the body. It has a honeycomb-like structure and carries a charge that allows it to capture toxins and escort them out of the body. At the same time it is inert and therefore does not react chemically with food or body fluids. Zeolite powder removes heavy metals, for example lead, cadmium, aluminium, arsenic and mercury and also radioactive metals. In this way it also reduces the load on the liver, so helps remove pesticides, herbicides and dioxins, and reduce the viral load. It helps buffer blood sugar levels, improves nutrient absorption, promotes healthy gut flora, reduces allergic reactions, enhances the immune system, and generally help prevent premature ageing. Zeolite agrees with many people who do not get on with other clays.

Thinking about the situation of radioactive toxicity in the world at large there are a number of strategies we need to take. Zeolites will take out heavy metals including radioactive fallout. Radioactive iodine is another matter. Our protection here is to have our own natural iodine levels well up, by supplementation, preferably with nascent iodine. Unfortunately, due to soil depletion, we no longer get enough from food. Sea vegetables, especially kelp, are the best food sources but probably not enough. Fluoride and chlorine are not good for our bodies but have a similar atomic structure to iodine (they are all in a chemical group called halogens) and are lapped up by the body readily when you are deficient in iodine. So is radioactive iodine. Iodine is needed by every gland of the body, especially the thyroid gland and pineal. It is crucial for the growing unborn child's intelligence too. The sense in supplementing with it is obvious.

MSM and the Beauty Mineral Sulphur

MSM or methyl sulfonyl methane is a nutritional from of sulphur, one of the most important elements to the body. MSM is the form of sulphur that is easiest for us to assimilate. In nature it is made by algae in the sea and is taken up into the clouds by evaporation. It then reaches the water courses and plants through the rain. Modern food processing, storage and washing of food means that most of it is lost and supplementation can be very beneficial. Supplements come in the form of a white powder or tablets and are generally made from plant material of some kind, wood or fossil material. They are naturally taken with water. MSM softens the cell walls which means that nutrients enter and toxins can leave more easily. This is why it is so often included as part of cleansing protocols. Sulphur is often described as a beauty mineral. It improves hair texture and can actually increase waviness of hair which depends on sulphur bonds. It softens skins, heals scar tissue and helps build collagen when taken with a source of vitamin C . It is good for joints, increases body flexibility and can reduce pain and inflammation. It can combine with heavy metals in the body such as lead, mercury and cadmium and escort them out of the body. Conversely these metals can lap up sulphur creating a shortage in the body.

Take about ½ to 1 teaspoon twice a day with water, rising to 1 tablespoon as necessary.

CoQ10 and Ubiquinol

CoQ10 is an enzyme needed for the mitochondria in the cells of our bodies to make energy. In our youth our bodies make their own supply. As we grow older we need to take it in from outside sources. The only food group with appreciable sources is organ meats which we may choose not to eat for a variety of reasons. Ubiquinol is the form that it is possibly easier for the body to use. I always mention this supplement to people past their thirties because I know the enormous benefits it can bring, restoring energy levels from years back for example in terms of walking speeds.

Telomerase Activators and Longevity

With the advent of stem cell therapy to actually rebuild tissue, telomerase activates to protect DNA, and bio-identical hormones that can enable the DNA to be read the way it's designed to be, we potentially have huge advances to be made in anti-ageing. The simple truth is that we are not meant to age as fast as we do. If you think about it, children of late puberty age are bright and capable, and they are not ageing. The implications are huge and far reaching. If we fix the glitch, which is possible, then these measures won't even be necessary. It is a reassuring thought that we have essentially the same DNA in later years as we did as children. If we can just hang onto it and avoid it being damaged then we may have all kinds of things in store for us including reaching a very old age with long term health. Wouldn't it be wonderful to combine the wisdom of age with the youthfulness of the young? This situation existed in the past and can exist again.

It seems that part of this anomalous situation we are in, part of the glitch, is that an important enzyme, telomerase is inactive, not present or switched off. So what does this mean? In short, telomerase is an enzyme that lengthens telomeres, the end of chromosomes that prevent damage to our genetic material. If telomerase is present in our bodies our genetic material is preserved for longer. Astragaloside IV otherwise known as TA65 is a telomerase activator extracted from the root of the plant astragalus. It is only found in a very small percentage of the roots. In time more plants containing telomerase activators are likely to be confirmed.

For the moment this supplement is having demonstrable results, effecting many people's health for the better and giving them more energy. This supplement is expensive, but more affordable versions are coming onto the marketplace and if you can afford it is worth considering.

Here's a more detailed description of what is going on, if it interests you. To me this is fascinating. The word telomere comes from the Greek 'telos' meaning 'end' and 'mere' meaning 'part'. The function of telomeres is a necessary part of chromosome replication. They are the tiny segments located on the end of each chromosome. They prevent damage to our genetic material by letting their extremities shorten during the process of cell replication and division. If we did not have telomeres the chromosomes of our cells could possibly become undifferentiated and fuse together causing abnormalities and mutations that could potentially lead to serious problems. Telomeres have been likened to the plastic bits on the end of a shoelace that are called aglets. Once they degrade to a point where they break apart the shoelace easily can unravel and usually does. When our telomeres become too short a whole cascade of degenerative diseases that are associated with ageing occur. Basically the cells with the shortest telomeres are going into old age (senescence). At this point they are near to the end of their lives (apoptosis) which unfortunately can often lead to a lot of collateral damage to other cells.

In 1961 it was concluded by Dr Leonard Hayflick that there is a finite limit to the amount of times a cell can replicate. This is known as the Hayflick limit. Previously it was believed that normal body cells were potentially immortal.

Hayflick subsequently concluded that if humans optimised their epigenetic potential, in other words have an ideal diet, living environment, exercise, low stress etc we can live for around 120 to 130 years! This is the typical lifespan of people living in ideal situations such the Hunza and Villcabamba. Now we understand the links between the Hayflick limit and telomeres. When the telomeres become too short or non-existent the cells can no longer successfully divide. In other words there is a finite amount of length on our telomeres before we start to witness the diseases associated with old age.

When we are conceived we have about 15,000 base pairs (building blocks in our DNA) This not many considering the chromosome can have approx 240 million base pairs. By the time we are born we have burned through about a third of them so now we are down to ten thousand. Our lifetime generally burns through about another five thousand until we get down to the last five thousand. This is the point at which old age and most of the pathological conditions associated with old age set in.The protective material on our DNA is getting lost as our cells divide.

About a decade ago that telomeres were discovered. It was found that the ends of the DNA molecular strands had a long series of meaningless code ("TTAGGG" in the language of DNA enzymes) that kept repeating and repeating. It was noticed that these strands, called telomeres, were longer in young cells (about 10,000 base pairs) and shorter in older cells (about 5,000 base pairs). When the telomeres got too short, the cell died. In 1973, a Russian biologist named Alexey Olovnikov was the first to recognise the issue of telomere shortening and subsequently predicted the existence of telomerase and came up with the original telomere hypothesis of ageing and how telomere health directly relates to cancer.

Telomerase is an enzyme that was discovered in 1984 by Elizabeth Blackburn and Carol Grieder at the University of California, Berkeley. It is a ribonucleoprotein that adds length to telomeres. Undifferentiated sperm cells for example divide millions of times and their telomeres never get short. This is the reason why a 90 year old man can still father children. Telomerase is also present in embryonic stem cells. It appears that when cells differentiate, for example go from being a stem cell to being a heart cell or a lung cell, then telomerase becomes dormant. If you would love to extend your lifespan while at the same time maintaining your body tissues finally there is now a solution to this issue.

Astragaloside IV is the world's first proven telomerase activator, although there are probably many. It is found in a certain subset and species of astragalus roots. TA-65 is an increasingly popular supplement made from astragaloside IV. Ron Teeguarden's super pill 2 sold by Dragon Herbs is another option. When a telomerase activator such as astragaloside IV is taken daily it turns on the hTERT gene which activates the enzyme telomerase and so in this way you can lengthen your telomeres. You can be tested to measure your telomeres before, during and after taking a telomerase activator to show actual changes in telomere length. However, long before any increase in telomere length can be measured, significant other changes are likely to be noticed. Examples of benefits reported by people taking telomerase activators are: increased energy and vitality, glowing skin, improvements to hair and nails, increased sexual energy, increased ability to focus mentally, improved memory and improved vision. In tests there have been statistically significant changes including: improved immune system, increased bone density, improvements in blood pressure, cholesterol and insulin levels. Hundreds of people have used telomerase activators since 2005 with no adverse effects reported.

I get the feeling and impression that telomerase is actually doing something more than just lengthening telomeres, amazing and important as this is in itself. I get the feeling that this enzyme, like most biochemical substances in the body has multiple purposes. The experience of being on a telomerase activator is quite distinct. It is a feeling of changing your life trajectory. This is more than increasing lifespan. It is about turning on an enzyme that we have not experienced since we were embryonic. Some people have reported that they feel as if they are breaking out of a shell and that they feel an ever increasing passion for life. The surge of energy for some people at times feels like a kundalini experience. One of the most significant effects we have noticed is that we actually feel more. There is a feeling of living a life of living rather than dying, a particular experience way beyond the explanations given. This has to be a good thing. We are beginning to defy cultural death programming. That is not to saying we are immortal, rather that we could regain our natural healthy lifespan and die more gracefully.

There are several suspected telomerase activator already. There are probably many foods that activate telomerase but as of yet none of them are proven, suspected foods are things like purslane, certain medicinal mushrooms, haritaki (part of the Ayurvedic Triphala/three fruits formulation), pharmaceutical grade fish oil and the amino acid supplement carnosine. It remains a very interesting topic and we will see how this story unfolds.

Astaxanthin

A brief mention here of one of the most powerful antioxidants discovered, it is remarkable in that it is soluble in fat, which enables it to be carried to particular tissues that it is difficult for other antioxidants to reach in the body. It has a reputed ability to slow down macular degeneration in the eyes.

ASEA

A relatively new supplement this product is said to contain stabilised redox signalling molecules. These molecules are essential to cell processes and diminish from the age of puberty. They are crucial to the carrying of information within the body and orchestrating tissue regeneration. People are experiencing noticeable results with it, in many ways.

Specially For Women

Progesterone Cream

Due to the anomalous hormonal situation we are currently in, the balance of oestrogen compared to progesterone in most women is too high. This is an increasing problem even for young women and as women go through the years, this imbalance, or 'oestrogen dominance', tends to get more extreme.
To further compound things, in modern times we have the arrival of oestrogen mimicers, xenoestrogens, in chemicals in our environment, including plastics. I go more into this later. I recommend using a reputable natural progesterone cream. By rubbing a tiny amount onto varying fatty areas of the body for half the days of the cycle, progesterone levels are gradually restored.

Pregnenolone

Pregnenolone is the precursor of all the sex hormones and lowers as we grow older. It is a nootropic i.e. it improves brain function. Some people feel benefit from it, others don't get on with it, it's a matter of trying it to see. Benefits can include alleviation of menstrual and menopausal symptoms, improved cognitive function and memory, reduced anxiety and reduction in joint pain.

Evening Primrose Oil and Deer Antler

These can both help relieve menopausal symptoms such as hot flashes. Deer antler should be from antlers that have been naturally shed.

Dong Quai

Dong quai, Angelica sinensis, also known as the "female ginseng," is a fragrant plant with a cluster of small white flowers. The flower belongs to the same botanical family as carrots and celery. People in China, Korea, and Japan dry its root for medicinal use. Dong quai has been used as an herbal medication for more than 2,000 years. It has been appreciated by many women for its help with menstruation, menopause and fertility. It regulates oestrogen levels, is a blood tonic, helps blood circulation and is calming. It also can provide relief for inflammation, heart disease and other diseases, though there are some contraindications for some illnesses.

There's a wonderful formula from Dragon Herbs, called Magu's secret which contains Dang quai root, along with Schizandra fruit, Goji berries, Chinese White Peony root, Codonopsis root, Cynomorium stem, and Longan fruit.

Rhodiolla

I have mentioned rhodiolla earlier. Here I want to share its value in terms of helping women going through the hormonal changes of menopause avoid common problems like forgetfulness and emotional swings during this time. It seems ti fill in some of the gaps caused by lowering oestrogen levels without causing the problems of hormone replacement therapy.

Specially for Vegans but can apply to all

As we went into earlier, to continue successfully with a 100% plant based diet through the years, well chosen supplements can make all the difference. Why is this? The plant foods we buy in stores are a far cry from those we would forage in our natural forest biological home, where soil and insect material and so on would inevitably be part of the diet. Also, of course we are not always exposed to enough sunshine to get the vitamin D we need. D3 is not available from plant foods and UVB rays from sunshine is not available to all of us all year round. The basic list to make sure you are covered is vitamin D3, K2 or a copious amount of greens and fermented foods, B12, for women - iron, a good EPA and DHA algae omega 3 supplement, possibly vitamin A in retinol form (be careful about the brand and quantity you use as vitamin A can be toxic in too large a dose).

Vitamin D

I highlighted vitamin D under vegan supplements because it is a fat soluble vitamin and the traditional food source is animal fats. It is in fact a hormone which affects the functioning Of the entire body. It has come to be described as the happiness hormone, needed for good mood, and in substantial doses is having massive impact on individual's health and sense of wellbeing. It is important in the assimilation of some minerals, such as calcium. Vitamin D mega-dosing is becoming increasingly popular. After all we are designed to live in the tropics where we would receive far more sunshine than we do in temperate latitudes. There are arguments for and against vitamin D mega-dosing. If you do it, it is essential to ensure that you also take in sufficient vitamin K2 either through supplements or fermented foods. You can read more details in Jeff Bowle's book on the subject listed in the references.

The plant form D2 is not the same as D3 which we need. I will expand on this because it is deficient in so many people, vegan or not, and there are some facts behind this that I think people need to know about. Ideally we make it in our skin from sunshine, but for people in temperate latitudes this simply won't happen for much of the year.

There is a 'vitamin D' winter if we live a long way from the equator; the length of this winter depends on the exact latitude. There is an article in the references which goes into this in more detail. In Britain it is from approximately September to March. The latitude determines the angle at which the sun's rays reach us and therefore the amount of UVB radiation we receive. It is UVB rays that create vitamin D3 in the skin. Areas of the world where this is an issue include the south of South America, South Australia, New Zealand, North America and Europe. In the tropics there is enough sunshine if you go out of doors with bare skin sufficiently.

Vitamin D is fat soluble, and if we are not taking on vitamin D through sunlight it needs to be taken with fat in order to be properly absorbed. There are two common types of vitamin D: Vitamin D3 (cholecalciferol) and Vitamin D2 (ergocalciferol). We need vitamin D3 rather than vitamin D2. You can obtain soft gel D3 supplements, drops and sprays. The richest food sources include fermented fish liver oil, butter (preferably raw) and high vitamin butter oil.

Another option is tanning beds or sun-showers which provide UVB for vitamin D and tanning without the UVA which damages skin. After exposure to UVB rays, make sure you wait as many hours as you can before showering. Why? After UV exposure, your skin produces a powdery substance that is then absorbed into the skin and converted to vitamin D by the body. If you wash this off too early, you interfere with the amount of vitamin D made.

By the way, when people begin to eat larger quantities of fresh raw fruit and vegetables they invariably report that their skin improves it's tone and responds better to sunshine, being less likely to burn and more likely to evenly tan.

Vitamin D is a happiness hormone which is also essential for health in many ways. Vitamin D activates the immune system: with vitamin D in the bloodstream, T cells become "armed" and begin seeking out invaders that are then destroyed and carried out of the body.

While minerals are the basic elements of matter, needed to build our bodies, vitamins are needed to take them to where they need to go. Vitamin D is needed to make sure that calcium goes to where it needs to go in the body while vitamin K2 is needed to enable vitamin D3 to do its job in this way.

The Vitamin B Complex

This is one of the most important groups of nutrients for mental health. It includes B1, B2, B3, B5, B6, B8, B9, B12, B15 and B17. I recommend taking a B complex supplement including B12. A dip in the intakes of any member of the B group will cause problems and fast. B vitamins are water soluble and pass out of the body quickly. Combining supplementing with good diet can equally cause spectacular results. They help promote good sleep.

- Vitamin B1 (thiamine) is needed for energy production, its deficiency leads to beriberi. Thiamine helps carry lead out of the body
- Vitamin B2 (riboflavin) is needed in body growth, repair and cell respiration. It helps maintain the health of the nervous system, the assimilation of iron and, along with Vitamin A, great vision.
- Vitamin B3 (niacin) deficiency causes depression and psychosis. Sometimes supplementation is used to help with mental problems. Those taking B3 niacin for the first time should exercise caution by commencing with a dosage not exceeding 200 mg and drinking plenty of water.
- Niacin is used in fat cell cleanses as part of a specific protocol (covered further in a Chapter 7).

Vitamin B5 (pantothenic acid) is believed to possibly improve memory, learning, and cognitive abilities.

Vitamin B6 (pyridoxine) is essential for making neurotransmitters. It converts amino acids into serotonin, a deficiency of which brings on irritability, violence, poor memory and a dive in overall cognitive and social performance.

Vitamin B7 (biotin) is known as the energy and beauty nutrient and assists our cells' mitochondria in producing the energy molecule adenosine-triphosphate (ATP). Biotin is used in the transformation of consumed carbohydrates, fats and proteins into energy, which is then stored in the liver and muscle tissue in the form of glycogen. Glycogen, when needed, is released from these stores and readily converted into glucose, which the body then chemically 'burns' as a fuel to produce physical energy. Biotin catalyses many enzymatic reactions in the body.

Vitamin B8, Inositol is a B nutrient used to treat mental mental disorders, panic attacks and anxieties.

Vitamin B9 (folic acid) works in conjunction with B12. It is well known in helping to avoid birth defects, such as spina bifida and neural tube defects. It is essential for oxygen delivery to the brain. A deficiency in either causes anaemia. Ideal supplementation for folic acid is around 400 mcg daily.

PABA or paraaminobenzoic acid, is a component of B9 (folic acid) and acts as a co-enzyme in the body. It assists other B vitamins in making red blood cells, metabolising proteins, and helping with skin disorders.

Vitamin B12 (methylcyanocobalamin) has been shown to improve the rate at which rats learn. Lack of B12 leads to anaemia, confusion and poor memory. Methylcobalamin is the most effective form of B12 supplementation. Therapeutic dosage is between 500 – 1,000 mcg a day.

Vitamin B15 (pangamic acid) has been described as 'instant oxygen' and has been used by Russian athletes for years to gain a competitive edge. Almost all research into this nutrient has come from Russia. Pangamic acid has been described as capable of delivering "flashy brilliance" to orgasms.

Choline is described as part of the B complex and is the base ingredient of lecithin. It helps in the formation of the 'memory' neurotransmitter molecule, acetylcholine.

Vitamin B17 (Laetrile or amygdalin) is often referred to as the anti-cancer vitamin. Like B15, this nutrient has been clouded with controversy.

So what's the story with B17. Well, these days it's hard to know what to believe, but there's something about this that rings true and there are plenty of reports of its efficacy. Vitamin B17 is among the main components of food in cultures like Hunzas, Eskimos, Abkasians etc. and these tribes have never ever reported a cancer case. Biochemist Dr. Ernst Krebs was instrumental in bringing B17 to the modern world and you can read more about his work online. In any case, including the foods mentioned is a good step all round. The story about vitamin B17, otherwise known as laetrile, nitroloside or amygdalin is fascinating so I will give it some space here.

Vitamin B17 is a name used to describe a large group of water-soluble, non-toxic, sugary, compounds found in over 800 plants, many of which are edible. The theory goes that cancer, although caused by many factors, is at root a metabolic disease, a disease of lack of nutrition, in a similar way that scurvy is a metabolic disease caused by lack of vitamin C. In this case the nutrient in question is B17. When part of the body is damaged in some way stem cells rebuild the damaged area, it's as if there are little 'cancers' forming regularly in the body. If this healing process is not halted in timely manner when it is complete, then the growth can get out of hand and become a tumour and cancer diagnosed. It is thought that nitrilosides, through their cyanide and benzene breakdown products, halt the stem cell healing process in the necessary way. Nitrilosides comprise of molecules made of natural sugar, hydrogen cyanide, and a benzene ring or an acetone. though the intact molecule is non-toxic and does not harm normal cells. Cancer cells love sugar. They eat the sugar and in the process releases cyanide, which only attacks cancer cells. When laetrile and the enzyme beta-glucosidase come in contact, laetrile breaks down to 1 molecule of HCN, 1 molecule of benzaldehyde and 2 molecules of glucose. Only the cancer cells in the body contain this enzyme.The logic is simple. HCN must be manufactured and shouldn't be freely floating around. If there are no cancer cells in the body, HCN will not be formed as there is no beta-glucosidase.

There is plenty of precedent for believing that a once fatal disease could turn out simply to be a metabolic disorder. At one time the metabolic disease scurvy killed hundreds of thousands of people, sometimes entire populations. It found total prevention and cure in the ascorbic acid or vitamin C component of fruits and vegetables. Similarly, the once fatal diseases pernicious anaemia, pellagra, beri beri, countless neuropathies, and the like, found complete cure and prevention in specific dietary factors, that is, essential nutrients in an adequate diet. Before these diseases were understood, before the means of total prevention and cure were discovered, it was widely believed that these dietary deficiency diseases were due to viruses, bacteria, bad air, infection, or some such cause.

In the past, human diets were rich in nitrilosides, but the modern processed diet can easily be almost completely lacking in them. For example, the nitriloside rich cereal millet was once more widely used in human nutrition than wheat, which, being a highly hybridised grain, contains no vitamin B17. B17 was present in everyone's diet until the industrial revolution because it was in some of the seeds and grains that were used to make bread, as well as of course it being consumed in other foods. During industrialisation, bread making was simplified as a commercial process and bread began to be made from just wheat, . Vitamin B17 appears in abundance in untamed nature. B17 is bitter to the taste and humans taste buds have changed over time due to a deviation away from a natural diet. In an attempt to improve tastes and flavours, we humans have eliminated bitter substances like B17 by selection and cross-breeding. However many of the foods that have been domesticated still contain the vitamin B17 in that part not eaten by modern humans, such as the seeds in apricots.

The following foods contain appreciable amounts of B17:

1. Seeds of Fruits or Kernels: These have the high concentrations of B17, second only to bitter almonds. Seeds of apricot, cherry, apple, peach, nectarine, plum, pear and prune contain good amounts of laetrile.
 2. Nuts: including macadamia, bitter almond and walnuts.
3. Beans: Burma, broad (vicia faba), lentils (sprouted), mung (sprouted), lima, scarlet runner, rangoon.
4. Berries: Nearly all wild berries for example chokeberry, blackberry, Christmas berry, elderberry, raspberry, cranberry, strawberry.
5. Grasses: acacia, aquatic, alfalfa (sprouted), milkweed, Sudan, minus, white clover, wheat grass.
6.Seeds: Flax, Chia, Sesame.

There are more references for this material at the end of the book. Listed in the Appendices is an evaluation of some of the more common foods.

Vitamin C

Vitamin C is another water soluble vitamin which we need to take in every day. Major deficiency used to cause scurvy but lesser deficiency may be implicated in modern illnesses such as heart disease. It so needed to form collagen. The large amount of fresh fruit and vegetables that we should ideally be consuming should in theory address most of our needs.

However as vitamin C is in the frontline for dealing with environmental toxicity we may need to supplement. It's wise to choose the brand carefully as many versions these days are made from GMO corn.

Tonic Herbs

Tonic herbs are those which can be taken ongoingly day after day. It's truly magical the effects that tonic herbs can have on the way you feel and your ability to function in the world. Some of my favourite herbs are, ginkgo, rhodiolla, schizandra, Siberian ginseng, tulsi and he shou wu. Ginkgo improves blood flow, including to the brain and enhances cognition and memory. Rhodiolla is an all round tonic, good for many things. It is especially useful for engendering mental alertness as an alternative to caffeine, for work or pleasure. Rhodiolla, schizandra, and Siberian ginseng is a particularly powerful combination and is the basis of the Diamond Mind formulation by Dragon Herbs. This combination can help protect mental function in seniors but is useful to optimise mental performance in younger people too.Tulsi can help relive stress amongst other things. The medicinal mushroom lion's mane is mentally activating and rebuilds neural tissue. It is particularly useful after periods of stress or malnutrition, as stress and malnutrition have the opposite effect.. Then we are beginning to get into the realm of brain biochemical supplementation or nootropics and we move into the next chapter.

I think of neuroactive nutrition in terms of layers. The macronutrition consisting of fruits and vegetables, leaves, roots, seeds etc. Then the superfoods, fermented foods, raw dairy etc. Supplements and mild tonic herbs that boost brain chemistry get added in on top. Then those powerful herbs and supplements that are taken in small quantities yet make substantial adjustments to the way we feel and=[- the perspective point of our consciousness. This is the next chapter.

5. Brain Biochemicals to Optimise Potential

This is the next layer. After bringing in the building block nutrition and tonic herbs we can tweak our systems still further and begin to kick start archaic systems within that enable us to run at our full potential and get that sense of connection that we innately know is possible. We can awaken more of our human genius and capacity for cognitive ecstasy, wonder and awe; that feel good factor that is impossible to fully describe – yet we know when we feel it, simply because it feels so right and natural. The revelations in this chapter are unique in that they are based on the deep understanding of the biochemistry of the human condition and origins revealed in the research spelled out Tony Wright. I have had the opportunity to discuss with many people the results they have experienced using these methods and they are pretty consistent.

It may be that many of humanity's spiritual teachers have been fortunate enough to have particularly good brain biochemistry and so are naturally more tuned into exalted states. Advice along the lines of telling people to feel more love may be as helpful to the rest of us as a cheetah telling a tortoise to run faster. We may genuinely need biochemical help to restore our brain function to a level where it can feel more, and the states of consciousness described by various teachings become reachable. As already mentioned, our pineal glands are currently under producing some key biochemicals. We are at a stage as humans where we need specific neurotransmitter/hormone supplementation, in addition to our natural biological diet, to operate at our best.

When I first began exploring this subject it was not talked about much. Now, thankfully there is a wave of interest in nootropics, micro-dosing and so forth. I call the combination of undamaged fatty acids, undamaged amino acids, fruit compounds, tonic herbs and nootropic herbs, Neuroactive Nutrition. It is nutrition that can boost our neural chemistry so that we have an expanded and definitely more ecstatic experience of life. We are designed to live in a state of what could be called cognitive ecstasy. This is not a state of being 'out of it', but a state of being exceptionally grounded, aware, inspired, creative, relaxed and energised. A state of true intelligence and being connected and sensitive to the forces of nature. We feel more and, as we have seen, true feeling is our natural guidance system, our way of self correcting, knowing where we are going and what is good. Feeling is the life force at work in us.

As we have seen in the human story, it is just a glitch, an anomaly in our situation that we are not experiencing this level of connection as a matter of course. Rebuilding and nourishing our neural systems, fuelling them and restoring archaic biochemistry is possible using a fusion of ancient and modern wisdom. This is plant medicine at work, restoring our connection to the plant realm is our healing. The chemicals that are so often used to attempt this reconnection are invariably from plant sources. As humans, we simply long for these states, and the sense of connection with the source of our lives. There are healthy sustainable ways to establish this sense of a natural high. On a clean natural diet we are already half way there.

Through major experiences with entheogenic plant medicines, people experience great revelations about who they are, what life is about, the nature of reality, and most of all that there is more to life than what is thought of as the normal state of consciousness and the values that go with it. Entheogen means "generating the divine within"(entheos is Greek for inspired; gen is Greek for producing) The term was coined in 1979 as a respectful term for plant chemicals that are ingested to induce a 'non-ordinary' state of consciousness, a state of divine inspiration. Entheagen is the feminine version of the word I came across which acknowledges the incredible femininity of the planet we live on (in scientific terms it is negatively charged with electrons) and the power of feminine healing. The word enthusiasm has the same roots. Enthusiasm

is such a liberator. Experiencing even our most trying emotions enthusiastically liberates us from them into a state of enthusiasm.
Profoundly deep plant medicine experiences have changed people's perception of life. They 'break open the head' so that the bigger realms are glimpsed. In brain terms we are talking about major right brain experiences. In fact it has be shown that plant medicines activate the right hemisphere, not the left. When they are taken with the base line of the nutrition described here, they can have an exceptionally pure quality without the extraneous material linked to artificial diet. A sense of being beyond death is a sign of opening up to layers of reality not perceived in left hemisphere dominated reality; one that might have been routine for our ancestors. The usual sense of self is relegated to the sidelines and happily so!

Combining these experiments with sleep deprivation to calm the left hemisphere has opened new windows for researchers in this area, even extraordinary senses of being awake that we do not normally experience, in everyday life, even a sense of being awake in the dream. This is well beyond any intellectual 'realisation'. Natural diet, neuroactive nutrition and sleep deprivation combined is one of the most powerful ongoing shamanic practices available to us in these times. The left hemisphere gets tired more quickly than the right and if the right hemisphere is well nourished its perception can shine through and the lens of consciousness can become a little clearer for a window of time. Eating a predominantly nutrient rich raw diet lessens the need for sleep for most people. So there's a double impact; the right brain gets nourished, while the left hemisphere dominance is reduced.

It has been tempting for people to come back from these experiences with a great revelation to change the way they run their lives, but this is really missing the point. Ideally people benefit from an ongoing sense of this connection from right hemisphere and pineal activation that informs and inspires every aspect of their lives. This is a state that can feel normal functional and familiar. I state here clearly that I cannot make any recommendations because this work is strictly experimental also people need to be aware of laws wherever they are. Ultimately, the idea is to reactivate right hemisphere or whole brain awareness and pineal function, and then eat our natural biological diet and live a natural lifestyle. Then we would experience this sense of connection. It takes researchers to do these experiments, as what is experienced in heightened awareness cannot be deduced by left brain logic.

Firstly I'll talk about the biochemistry that was originally supplied by the pineal gland then we'll look at traditional solutions and what we can do today.

In Chapter 2, talking about the human story I described how the pineal gland is actually designed to pump much greater amounts of melatonin than it does today and also monamine oxidase inhibitors, which keep neurotransmitter levels up and also tiny tiny amounts of DMT (dimethyltryptamine) which is in fact an essential neurotransmitter which enables us to see patterns both visually and mentally.

So we have the question of how to maintain this biochemistry in a safe and healthy way. Sometimes experimenters wonder whether supplementing will somehow get them 'used to' these biochemicals so they will not work any more. I would answer that these substances are required for optimal functioning, that we no longer make them in sufficient quantities, and we need them. The intention is to kick start the pineal into producing its own hormones again and get the whole feedback loop going in a positive direction. Reports I have heard indicate that this kind of supplementation does not lead to dependence, rather the opposite.

The challenge is to judiciously supplement with the deficient biochemicals such as melatonin, monoamine oxidase inhibitors and possibly tiny amounts of dimethyltryptamine in its natural plant form to restore a more conducive brain chemistry. Of course I am not talking about dimethyltryptamine isolated, I am talking about it in the form it exists in all living beings and particularly in some plants. There are many countries in the world where it is legal to use these plants, in the traditional way.

Melatonin is increasingly becoming known for its anti-ageing, immune boosting and antioxidant qualities. Also its ability to promote healthy sleeping patterns and protect us from electromagnetic pollution. When people begin to supplement with melatonin, many report feeling calmer and also having increased feeling and empathy, leading to more harmonious relationships between family members and friends.

Melatonin levels can be boosted quite simply with supplements. Start with 1mg a night and progress upwards from there at a rate you feel comfortable with. There are even some low dose melatonin supplements made with grasses. Initially you may feel groggy in the morning – this is due to an excess of melatonin receptors resulting from long term deficiency - this will pass. Take melatonin at bedtime and certainly not before driving or using heavy machinery. Although it was once abundant in our brains, we are now unused to operating in the meditative state it promotes. Melatonin rich foods include montmorency cherries and grasses such as wheat grass and barley grass. Festuca arundinacea grass has one of the highest melatonin contents of any plant and is native to the British Isles.

Monoamine Oxidase Inhibitors

Now we come to pinoline, the MAOI or mono-amine oxidase inhibitor which is naturally secreted by the pineal gland. Monoamine oxidase is a class of enzymes which break down certain neurotransmitters. When MAOI's or monoamine oxidase inhibitors are introduced these enzymes are inhibited and the neurotransmitter levels go up. One way to boost these levels is with 'Happy Tea'. This consists of passion flower, (which contains analogues of pinoline) mixed with St John's Wort. Don't drink more than three or four mugs a day of this tea. As with most herbs moderation is a good idea. MAOI's also occurs in raw cacao - one reason raw chocolate makes people feel good. Years ago MAOI's were prescribed as antidepressants. And with good reason, it's partly a lack of them that is depressing humanity in the first place. However their use was stopped because it gave a lot of responsibility to the patient to manage their lifestyles. MAOI's inhibit the enzymes which digest tyramine rich foods such as animal products including dairy, fermented products, and soy products, so it is unsafe to consume them in the same digestive time window. There is a full list of these foods in the Appendices.

Dimethyltryptamine

DMT operates as a neurotransmitter in the brain. It is necessary for optimal brain function and is still produced in significant quantities by the pineal gland during peak experiences. As I explained it helps us see patterns both visually and through inner perception. It regulates the spacing of monatomic elements in the brain. It is created in small amounts by the human body during normal metabolism and is in some natural food sources but is broken down by monoamine oxidase. If MAOI's are being consumed the DMT has more chance of staying in circulation and reaching the brain.

DMT has become a recreational high which people smoke or inject relatively large doses. This is not what we are talking about here. We are talking about the tiny amounts needed by the brain to function what is actually a normal way. We need it to perceive patterns. DMT exists in all living things. In some plants it exists in significant amounts, and these plants have been used traditionally as medicines. Of course DMT was originally secreted by our pineal glands from where it can be readily lapped up by the brain. If it is taken into the digestive system through eating and drinking then MAOI's are needed at the same time to stop it being immediately broken down. This is the biochemical basis of the ayahuasca traditions. Two herbs such as banisteriopsis caapi and psychotria viridis , sometimes together with the juice of an acid fruit such as lemons or oranges are boiled up for several hours, even days. The banisteriopsis contains plentiful supplies of MAOI's, the psychotria DMT. In this way DMT is introduced into the system. In a few countries ayahuasca herbs have become legally challenged but there are still many countries where the tradition is respected by government, for example in Central and South America. There has been a long standing tradition, for example amongst the Huichol of Mexico that good medicines (drugs) are brought in to counter the bad drugs. There are legal and safe ways to proceed.

I have been told many anecdotes of the micro-dosing carried out by people clear in their intent to awaken their consciousness. Methods include taking a tablespoonful of a weak brew of banisteriopsis and psychotria first thing in the morning. It may be wise not to consume large amounts of tyramine rich foods such as animal, dairy, soy or fermented products at the same time. These are the foods traditionally avoided when using large doses of ayahuasca. In the case of micro-dosing it is not so critical but still, being careful can avoid the risk of making one feel unwell. Although in large doses ayahuasca can produce very dramatic effects including visions and a substantially altered sense of perception, in these small doses it just wakens the brain up a little, enhancing mood, creativity, inspiration, visual perception, and practical effectiveness. People who have done this have reported very similar experiences, a feeling that it was easier to know what to do, to deal with various daily problems etc. Of course in some countries of the world it is still possible and legal to continue this practice. There are many ayahuasca analogues available. These are combinations of herbs which fulfil the same biochemical function.

Meditation also quietens the left side of the brain thereby allowing more right hemisphere function, and so can help boost levels of these crucial biochemicals. In chapter 8 are listed some of the key activities and lifestyle practices for calming the left hemisphere and boosting the right. In our current situation there is a lot to be said for lining the whole lot up - excellent diet, biochemical supplementation, meditative and natural lifestyle with techniques to boost right hemisphere activity.

Psylocibin

It's odd to reflect that at the time I was first writing this book psylocybin mushrooms were still legal within UK Law. Of course they still are in many places. After ingestion psylocybin breaks down to become psilocin and causes altered states of awareness. As I explained, I don't believe that psychoactive mushrooms are what gave humans their awareness and intelligence, rather that they were used later on in the story to stimulate a sense of perspective akin to what we would naturally have experienced in our forest diet. What I want to mention as interesting here is that the psilocin molecule is remarkable similar to the DMT molecule (see illustration) and there are comparisons that can be made between their effects. However psilocin is not broken down by digestive enzymes is sometimes described as orally active DMT. However the effects are not exactly the same and it is DMT that occurs naturally in humans.

Serotonin   Psilocin   N,N-Dimethyltryptamine (DMT)

My sense of things is, that if the pineal gland was pumping its regular tiny doses of DMT, it would be fulfilling the function that people use psilocybin micro-dosing for. Micro-dosing with psilocybin, i.e. taking a sub-perceptual dose - an amount too small to produce traditional psychedelic effects - has become popular with people from athletes to media professionals, intellectuals and Silicon Valley workers. It is found to improve visual and mental acuity, energy, response time, problem solving skills; it also can alleviate depression. It is not found to cause disruption. The legal status of psilocybin varies across the world.

The Miracle of Iboga

Even after years of healthy eating and living habits, and all kinds of self-help, people can still feel very stuck. It's like they reached a wall - even after working with potent plant medicines ceremonies. It seems that learning to feel more does not always make people feel better ; which is a reason people often continue to choose not to feel more. Ultimately feeling more encourages us to adjust our lifestyles so we feel, but the path can be complex and uncomfortable, and there are hidden blocks in the way.

It is solution thinking and focusing on desirable outcomes, that makes us feel better and gets us somewhere. Negative thinking serves no purpose except to make ourselves and the people around us miserable. Yet we can still slip into it. It seems that negative thinking is addictive. And knowing that it is an addiction makes you no more able to stop being addicted to it then you would be able to stop a chemical substance addiction. In fact it seems like chemical substances are in some involved, they are the bodies own chemicals and intervention of some kind is needed. And this is where the miracle of iboga comes in.

Over the years I had got to hear many reports of people who have experienced personal transformation through therapeutic use of the iboga plant. The iboga root has been used for as long as anyone can remember in Central Western Africa in the areas of Gabon and Cameroon, where it grows. It is used for healing and initiatory purposes.

The main active ingredient in iboga is called ibogaine although a complex combination of chemistry is involved when the whole root is used. In the early sixties it was discovered by accident that it has addiction interrupting properties and could break addiction to powerful substances even such as heroin and cocaine. Also it breaks the alcohol dependence cycle and interrupts many other addictions. What's more it seems to address the underlying issues and traumas, hence it is described as twenty years of psychotherapy in one night!

Afterwards many people report that it is very difficult to think a negative thought. The connection between the addiction interruption and the cessation of negative thinking struck me. The molecules of emotion in our bodies - the peptides - can be addictive. When people have been traumatised or habitually think negative or fearful thoughts, they get into an addictive cycle with their own peptides. The emotions, and the conditions that cause them, can even be passed from generation to generation, creating what we call ancestral trauma. No one might even remember why a whole nation, tribe or family are a certain way, but it can be caused by events that happened a long time ago. This is connected to what Wilhelm Reich called the Emotional Plague. Iboga or ibogaine can interrupt the addictive cycle of drugs. It can also interrupt the addictive cycle of the chemicals of emotion.

To break the addictive cycle of chemical drugs a so called 'flood dose' must be given. It needs to be accurately weighed so it is enough to break the chemical cycle and not too much to be dangerous. African healers, experienced with iboga, have their own ways of conducting iboga ceremonies. For the purposes of modern medics dealing with addiction, ibogaine is extracted from the iboga root so an exact amount can be weighed based on the patient's body weight. For therapeutic use for purely emotional issues, micro-dosing can be very powerful and the whole root, ground up can be used. Several countries have either banned iboga or restricted its distribution, as it has been lumped into the general drugs category which is ironic as it heals drug addition. There are still plenty of countries where it is completely legal though and treatment can be sought.

Many people have benefited from this process. People typically take 0.25g to 0.4g a day depending on their sensitivity. For some, a month of micro-dosing is enough; others continue for several months. It seems to reset people from lives of what is essentially cycles of repeated trauma, to live the lives they are truly here for. Sometimes we simply are not the people we thought we were. Of course even after dealing with trauma chemicals we still have the left brain right brain split and all that entails, but this kind of therapy takes us to a point where we can engage with whatever we need to do to deal with that. People report feeling more comfortable in themselves afterwards taking iboga. Another application, that is being researched at the time of writing, is the use of ibogaine in the treatment of Parkinson's. It seems so far that it alleviates the symptoms and rebuilds neural tissue.

With the way cleared we can move forward to the next part of the story.

6. Living in Beauty ~ Natural Lifestyle

Natural, ecological lifestyle is way deeper than using natural products, or even being in natural surroundings; it's the beauty of living according to your true nature. We can easily get the impression that beauty is somehow elitist because of the way it is culturally defined. Stepping out of the narcissistic codependence trap by engaging in the larger world of nature, we can find our own natures.

"The conventional notion of the self with which we have been raised and to which we have been conditioned by mainstream culture is being undermined. What Alan Watts called "the skin-encapsulated ego" and Gregory Bateson referred to as "the epistemological error of Occidental civilisation" is being unhinged, peeled off. It is being replaced by wider constructs of identity and self-interest by what you might call the ecological self or the eco-self, co-extensive with other beings and the life of our planet. It is what I will call "the greening of the self.'
The crisis that threatens our planet, whether seen from its military, ecological, or social aspect, derives from a dysfunctional and pathological notion of the self. It derives from a mistake about our place in the order of things. It is a delusion that the self is so separate and fragile that we must delineate and defend its boundaries, that it is so small and so needy that we must endlessly acquire and endlessly consume, and that it is so aloof that as individuals, corporations, nation-states, or species, we can be immune to what we do to other beings."'World as Lover, World as Self' - Joanna Macy, 1991.

One of the benefits of living naturally is feeling right in ourselves. Food is a very central and solid part of this because of the direct impact it has in our neurochemistry. Once that neurochemistry is happening we are going to feel an increasing sensitivity to nature in general and to our own natures.

Natural lifestyle is at one level natural food, homes, clothing, fresh water, ionisers and so forth. The deeper level that can be reached by doing these things is a sense of the beauty of life. This is when our senses get super-heightened. When we see the beauty we are moving into a supernatural state.

It is so important for our sense of belonging to be connected to living things that are bigger than ourselves - like trees, mountains and the stars, the sun, the wind and the rain. In so-called highly developed parts of the world humans have made themselves the biggest strongest living things in their environments and then ironically having chopped down trees and eradicated wild animals have brought in high rise buildings and motor vehicles to replace them. That causes a feeling of indescribable loneliness and neurosis, a failure to adapt to our environment. Even so, wherever we are we are on a living planet.

We still have the opportunity to connect to the life force, an organising, ordering influence. In other words it is syntropic. This is in contrast to the bare laws of physics which declare the universe to be moving into ever greater entropy or disorder. The golden mean, which I have referred to ,has been used classically to create works of art of great beauty. It is intricately encoded into the world of nature.

The first topic I am covering is earthing and electro-magnetics. Then I'll cover our relationship to time, exercise, sleep and the feeding of all our senses.

Earthing

Earthing or grounding has become a hot topic in recent times and many people are finding that long standing chronic ailments will almost magically disappear when they do this. Earthing is no more complicated than electrical connection to the Earth so that your voltage or frequency or electric field aligns with that of the Earth, and electricity from the Earth flows into you. You could think of it as natural electrical charging. Within the charge of the Earth our vibration is modulated so it is in harmony with the circadian rhythms of our environment. It can be done by walking barefoot on the earth or other skin contact with the Earth, Paddling or swimming in sea water is one of the most powerful earthing experiences because of the salt. Mineralised or salt water is much more conductive than pure water. Another way is use of equipment such as earthing sheets, throws, and earthing mats. Earthing sheets contain threads of silver which connect to a lead that is plugged into the earthing connection of a building or alternatively to a grounding rod that is put into the ground. There are also grounding shoes that enable you to walk in rough ground protected while still maintaining electrical connection.

Obviously we are designed to operate in electrical connection with the Earth. When homes were simpler and before people wore shoes with electrically insulating soles this was the norm. Humans were conceived, born, lived, and died in the bio-electromagnetic aura of the Earth. It's easy to give an example of how crucial this is to the body's workings. My favourite example is its role in metabolism. When we digest food and turn it into fuel this is an 'oxidative process'. A type of molecule called free radicals are produced. The way this is described in science is that they have an electron missing from the outer shells and are 'electron hungry', grabbing electrons from other molecules and causing a destructive chain reaction. 'Antioxidant' foods such as fruit and vegetables supply these electrons and prevent damage to the body. In our state of natural connection to the Earth electrons are naturally supplied and contribute to this so-called antioxidant effect.

Looking at the mental side of things, as our neural systems are electrical and the earth is electrical, it stands to reason that if you disrupt the natural electrical connection between the two it will have a negative impact. The Earth is the local source of our physical food and it is also our local source of electricity. If we cut the electric connection and then add in an artificial field of mains electricity, wifi, mobile signals and so forth, this will clearly affect our emotional and thought patterns, including our ideas of what we want. In our natural electrical field our desires are natural and healthy, they are for things that will actually fulfil us and bring happiness and are sustainable. On the more esoteric side of this subject we receive information and guidance in day to day living our lives through contact with the Earth. It is almost our original internet connection! Our desires become more health and life-affirming when we are immersed in the Earth's field rather than that of the artificial electric grid. Many years ago Fereydoon Batmanghelidj, in his book "The Body's Many Cries for Water", made known the crucial importance of drinking adequate water to the maintenance of basic health and prevention of disease. Now we are learning that 'earthing' is a similarly crucial requirement for health. The recommendation is at least 20 minutes earth connection twice a day for basic health needs. Personally I try maintain it most of the day one way or another. You can describe three levels of connection to the Earth: being in nature, immersing yourself in the bio-electromagnetic aura of the earth and playing your part in the Earth's story. We can tune into the planetary mind, using specific techniques. This is not 'channelling'. The Earth has an electromagnetic aspect to it like our own, Nowadays the idea of the Earth, sometimes known as Gaia having organising awareness has become familiar. Through observation of the lunar cycles and learning the story of the Earth, the connection can become increasingly and more consciously experienced. This is a specific art, innate and once natural to humans and needing to be rediscovered. We are designed to be wired into the bio-electromagnetic field of the Earth (BEMA). The challenge is to detect the messages we get and retain them, unelaborated with our own conditioning.

In addition to earthing equipment there are devices that will replicate a natural electrical field, neutralise the fields from wifi and mobiles and introduce so called 'negative ions' or electrons into the atmosphere, in a similar way to in nature.

The best devices I have come across so far is the Geocleanse, trademark of OEA (Orgone Effects Australia), available also at foodforconsciousness.co.uk. Everyone I have spoken to who has one has found a noticeable improvement in the feel of their home. The water energiser in this same product range negatively charges water in the way you would expect to find in flowing water in nature. Negative charge in this context is another way of saying electron rich. Negative ions are in abundance in natural environments and are beneficial to living things including ourselves. The thing to remember is that however much we minimise our own wifi and mobile usage, unless we are living in a relatively remote location, we are in the collective signal. Smart meters have an even more intense effect than either wifi or mobile masts and are now causing major health problems. You can learn more about this in the interview with Dr. Dietrich Klinghardt called Smart Meters & EMR - The Health Crisis Of Our Time, available on youtube.

Even if we do not have a smart meter installed in our own property we will be affected if our neighbours do. A geocleanse device can help protect us in his situation. The experience of the geocleanse I have seen so far has been remarkable and ironically you can end up with a more natural field in your own home that in the local countryside field. This is a strange quirk of the times we live in. be Earthing, by the way, increases melatonin levels and seems to give us more right hemisphere brain access.

Walking in Nature

Of course we all know that spending extended amounts of time in nature can take us to new heights of well-being. Walking in nature also has a psychological effect due to the effects of moving and looking into the distance and widens our mental horizons and sense that we can move forward in life. When we are walking we are focused on what is front of us whilst staying subliminally aware of what we are actually doing – in this way it resets us with good mental habits and clears our minds for inspiration. One of my quotations about human nature comes from Robert Lawlor who described humans as 'walking mystics'. "The human is the only organism wired so that walking is a spiralling motion opening up an imploding vortex of bioelectric field." When we walk we tap into energy and inspired thoughts that are difficult to access any other way.

Exercise and Fresh Air

Exercise affects our metabolism. It boosts endorphins, it's good for neurogenesis (brain regeneration) and this in itself boosts your mood. It helps us absorb tryptophan. There are eight essential amino acids, and tryptophan is one of them. Serotonin is made from tryptophan. The tryptophan molecule is a large one. If we have sedentary lives the other amino acids tend to be absorbed before the tryptophan. Carbohydrates help tryptophan be absorbed too. If we don't exercise there can be the tendency to eat extra carbohydrates. This is one of the body's many ways of protecting essential processes on the body. Obviously it would be better to exercise and if we snack on carbohydrates as a substitute for exercise this obviously can affect our health and weight. Another effect of exercise is through the lymphatic system. Like our blood, lymph fluid has a job to do of carrying around nutrients and removing toxins, but unlike blood it is not pumped around the body. It needs our movement in order to move. If we don't move our bodies frequently we are going to start feeling very sluggish. When we are under stress it is even more important to make sure we exercise. Stress hormones increase insulin levels and we are being chemically prepared for action. If we don't actually physically move then we mess up our body's chemical balance. Another mechanism by which exercise makes us feel better is that it increases endorphin levels. Exercise gets oxygen into us too. If we can do some of it in nature we are obviously going to feel the benefit of the fresh air. All in all exercise is so essential and so easily sidelined as not a priority.

A lot of people are resistant to exercise mainly because it is often looked upon as something that is to be tolerated and endured. This is mostly a mental block and is often based upon how we think things should be. A great approach is to choose a form of exercise that is fun for you and, rather than punishing yourself and telling yourself you have to go through some long drawn out ordeal. You can get a lot done in just 10 – 15 minute bursts which can be repeated several times a day . In fact this is the way children naturally exercise and is the best way to stimulate the production of human growth hormone, essential for not just growth of children but also the maintenance of our bodies. For some people this approach works very well but others may prefer the structure of a yoga class or a personal trainer. There are myriads of choices, for example walking, martial arts, bike riding, resistance exercise, yoga, weight lifting, running, gymnastics etc. Choose one or a combination that you can consistently apply and your emotional state is going to improve.

As time passes you may find that you get hooked on exercise and want to spend longer times at it. As we improve our lifestyles, our addictions and resistances have a tendency to be replaced by what could be described as an addiction to feeling better.

Fresh Living Water

Collecting natural living spring water is one of the most satisfying experiences. Of course these days we need to check that the source is not contaminated. Many springs are listed on findaspring.com. Collect water in glass or safe plastic bottles where possible. Many plastic bottles contain BPA (biphenol A) which is a hormone disrupter. You can obtain BPA free plastic bottles. Many people highly value distilled water. My concern is that it can strip minerals from the body and has lost its life force. While I keep an open mind on this subject I prefer natural living water. If there really is none local to you of course you can buy it in. Try to get it delivered in BPA free bottles.

Star Watching

Connecting to the stars and sky above is also an important part of our psychological health. Even the act of looking up lifts our mood. The patterns of the stars have a beneficial and informing impact on our psyches. The stars were our original source of guidance. Light pollution obscures their patterns in many places now. We have an innate sense that shimmering lights is where guidance comes from so we get drawn in instead to the shimmering lights of digital displays and so forth. The very fact that we are so attracted to these devices shows how natural it is to look at patterns of lights. The Earth too radiates light, which is is still possible for some people to see. Others can do so after a process of learning to do so using certain techniques. I believe that the ability to see this light, and receive guidance form it is part of our innate ability that can be rediscovered as we rebuild and reactivate our neural systems. This is the Holy Grail we seek. The sense of guidance we get from nature, such as the stars, birdsong and so forth is not in left brain language, but still can be decoded by our latent intelligence - increasingly so as we reactivate it. We start to have the experience of being activated by these signals from nature; this is sane and healthy and part of the way humans have lived for most of their existence. I know it is the opinion of some teachers and healers that star gazing and listening to birdsong helps activate our pineal glands and I suspect this is true.

Time

Our relationship to time is such a fundamental part of our lives that it would be easy to overlook as we think about natural lifestyle. We could view time as the most valuable resource in our lives. It's something we all have, and what we do with it determines our lives. Something I came to realise through studying real sky astrology is something I had already intuitively known. Each moment is unique, as unique as a snowflake. Each one has its own unique flavour. Moments come and go and we never experience the exact same moment again. How we act in these moments partially determines the degree to which we fulfil our destinies - the lives gifted to us. Or whether we merely fall into the hands of fate. Time and space are linked by natural rhythms and the more we tune into these the more we are able to accomplish and the more we are supported by the benign supernatural forces bigger than ourselves. Clock and calendar time are obviously something else. Most of us are obliged to engage with them for social reasons; somehow we need to weave the two systems together at this point, just as we weave the two hemispheres and two modes of being. Observing sunrises and sunsets when we can, following the phases of the moon and seasonal points through the year are a rational way of behaving. I think the effect on us of watching the sun rise is beyond what we can explain in left hemisphere language. Another cycle that is of great interest is the apsides of the moon, the movement of the moon towards and away from the earth which came into popular awareness at the time of the spring equinox supermoon of March 2011.

The cycles of human life are part of the study of celestial or real sky astrology. Conventional astrology is based on a theoretical sky twelve equal pizza slices or 'signs' each one correlated to a constellation in the sky. Because of an astronomical phenomenon called precession of the equinoxes these signs are no longer in the same place as the constellations they are named after. Added to which, the constellations are not of equal size but all completely different, as you would expect with natural objects.

There are eighty-eight constellations or distinct groups of stars to be seen in the sky. Thirteen of them lie on the path that the sun and moon travel on relative to our viewing position on Earth. These thirteen constellations are the ones referred to in Real sky astrology. Real sky astrology does not talk about personal psychology in the way that conventional astrology does, it is about the way we fulfil our destinies and the way we inherit our talents and passions from humanity that has gone before us. The patterns and codes are decoded in an expansive way so that the themes can enrich and fuel our lives. Discovering this way of looking at things has given many people a better sense of what their lives are about and a deep sense of fulfilment. Though this is an ancient science and art it has only been rediscovered in the last few decades.

Living Spaces

Our homes and workspaces have such a huge impact on our whole being. It is helpful to use natural materials as much as possible. Colours and décor are very important. Tastes can change when we change what we eat. The fractal structure of natural materials for our homes and clothing keeps us more connected to the life force.. Traditional materials like linen and hemp have a strong fractal structure. Fractals are the natural structure of living things, based on the Fibonacci series and Golden Ratio or Phi. It is used in art because it brings in a sense of beauty. It permeates the pattern of organic life. It is immensely helpful to fill our homes with the life force of plants, especially those that absorb pollution or provide us with food. Decluttering objects that belong to the past and have no place in our current reality frees us up energetically.

Sleep

Sleep is an interesting topic in the light of what we know about our condition. It seems that the left hemisphere needs more sleep than the right hemisphere and so sleep deprivation can be used as a tool for accessing right hemisphere function. This is why people so often get creative insights in the early hours of the morning. Experiments by Tony Wright and Steve Charter on sleep deprivation at Manchester Metropolitan University found that strength, dexterity and reaction times all improved on sleep deprivation combined with a nutritionally dense raw food diet. This was just one trial but there is much anecdotal evidence of people experiencing improved abilities when combining nutrient dense raw food diets with sleep deprivation. On the other hand, given that we are in a condition of left hemisphere cerebral dominance we do actually need sleep to function at our best and also maintain health. We really are in a dichotomy in this situation. For long term health and youth it seems that quality and quantity of sleep is essential for most people. Going to bed early at night and getting up early in the morning allows you to get the quality of sleep that is better before midnight. Much of our growth and tissue repair happens during our sleep. Early to bed and early to rise is the motto of many successful people. While we are sleeping the right hemisphere can be very active and we are refreshed by our dreams.

Periods of sleep deprivation do seem to have long term benefits though if handled properly, because of the right hemisphere access. Sleep deprivation is a shamanic practice not a healthy lifestyle practice. However the need for less sleep when eating a natural raw diet is genuine. It's as if you can get the benefits of both good sleep and mild reduction in duration of sleep. Our dream life can be much more active and beneficial if we sleep as far as possible outside artificial electrical fields such as mains electricity, wifi and mobile signals. Then we can connect into the electromagnetic filed of the Earth and beyond. This is where the Geocleanse can make such a difference in urban areas. The balance of work and exercise and sleep and relaxation is fundamental to well being.

Sleep has become a big issue because the artificial electromagnetic signals now flooding us, although not visible to us do reach and stimulate our pineal gland - which is sometimes known as the inner eye. When the light of the day fades this is supposed to be a signal to the pineal gland to start pumping more melatonin so that we sleep. If there are lots of high frequency waves which we cannot see they still enter the skull and are detected by the pineal gland and so melatonin production is not triggered in the same way. Of course our melatonin levels are too low already so the situation is compounded. As years go by our pineal glands tend to secrete less melatonin and supplementing at bedtime is a sensible health practice. You can read about this and get practical information about dosing in the "The Melatonin Miracle: Nature's Age-Reversing, Disease-Fighting, Sex-Enhancing Hormone" by Walter Pierpaoli. Earthing devices also increase melatonin levels though not as much as supplementation. Sleep well away from computers, phones and so forth.

Walking outside early in the morning and going to bed reasonably early at night aligns our circadian rhythms and can have miraculous effects on our happiness and productivity levels and is so often overlooked in the distractions of our 24/7 culture.

Warmth

With our tropical forest background we feel at our most relaxed when warm. When we are in cold environments we are stressed and it makes our minds work differently. At 24 to 28 degrees our bodies relax and our parasympathetic nervous system kicks in - so our minds work better as they are not focused on a perceived state of emergency.

Light and Colour, our Five Senses

Everything that goes into us affects our state. Light and colours are electromagnetic frequencies which affect how we feel, that's why colour therapy works. When people move into natural nutrition they often begin to gravitate towards the colours of nature. Bringing in warm azures, sunny yellows, vibrant greens and so forth change our mood. It's good to notice how the colours we use actually affect us because there is a tendency to choose colours which reinforce our temperaments. Natural sounds, smells and textures too make a difference. Our senses stimulate our right hemispheres and more expanded awareness. Incense has been used for millennia for this reason and it's known that frankincense lifts mood. Letting the sounds of nature, for example birdsong, the wind and rain, connects us to natural wisdom in a subtle but real way.

Loving and affectionate contact

Rapport with other humans who are committed to being real with each other and help us keep on track is a precious gift. Robert Lawlor talks about the days when from early childhood we were independent because we could obtain everything we needed from the natural environment. Then we were free to enjoy each other's company for the sake of kinship rather than as part of some survival strategy.

Eye connection is one of the most powerful tools for engaging the right hemisphere. And touch is even now being found to be a key factor in maintaining brain function as we grow older.

Disharmony with or loss of people in our lives is one of the most distressing experiences for most people. Conversely good relationships are one of the most important factors in human happiness. Some studies suggest they are the most important factor. Humans do seem to get on better when they are in the context of nature. In this situation their energy levels are naturally boosted and they are not trying to take so much energetically from each other. These days narcissism and codependence are big topics and I believe they arise from humans trying to have relationships with each other outside the context of the wider intelligence of nature. Healing comes though deep connection to the Earth and nature.

As I mentioned before, without the corresponding neurochemistry, it may be very difficult to experience feelings of love. Without feeling love just becomes another concept. In the current human condition the lack melatonin plays a part in this disconnection from feeling. As I described in Chapter, increasing melatonin levels tends to increase harmony between people. In fact being in the vicinity of parents and family members is known to increase melatonin levels in children. Watching television and computer screens decreases melatonin levels.

Empathy is the ability to feel in our own bodies what another person is feeling. In this state we don't generally wish people harm. In our most exalted state it may be impossible to deliberately and maliciously cause harm to any human, creature or living being. This is due to the extreme empathy and connection rather than a belief system. It is only because of our sense of separateness that we can behave in certain ways. In a state of empathy and connection our world grows bigger and we do not need to grow our ego to dominate it.

Retreats and Resets

Consistency is the key to success on this path. The different dietary and lifestyle choices weave together synergistically. Everyone gets off track at times. The important thing is that we can quickly get back on track. For example one formula is to connect into some natural stimulus such as birdsong, a walk in the woods or a swim in the sea - whatever is most immediately available. We also need to remind ourselves to focus our goals on what we truly want in life. And we need to physiologically and chemically reset. My reset recipes in this book are a brilliant way of getting food back on track. Posture too changes physiology and our thought patterns.

Retreats are a time to quieten the mind and go beyond language into dreaming. We can realign to natural cycles and establish healthy routines and rituals in our lives. They are times when we can focus on how we feel and polish our desires. Away from distraction we can focus on our purpose and the steps we need to take.

A long term personal goal is the setting up of a human research project where, away from the current culture, we can research what actually makes humans more functional, fulfilled and happy, using the material cited in this book as the starting point.

7. Cleansing and Regenerating your Body Ecology

The main theme of this chapter is that just as the Earth is an intelligent living entity and home to many species, we too are home to millions of microorganisms. We are an entire ecology and our intelligence is intricately connected to what is going on within it. Microbiome is the term that has come into use to describe this.

The Second Brain

It's quite a realisation that just as we are organisms living as a part of a much bigger living organism, planet Earth, and our own bodies are an entire ecology. In the middle of it all our own awareness juggles between macrocosmic forces, bigger than ourselves and microcosmic forces, those inside ourselves and our lives. Doing what we can to maintain a healthy inner terrain is part of this. Our neural systems and immune systems are connected to our inner ecology. The point of cleansing then is not purely inward looking but to clear our 'lens of consciousness' so we can experience the outer world in a more expanded way.

Recently the gut has become known as 'the second brain'. The part of the nervous system that controls the gastrointestinal system is sometimes called the enteric nervous system. Research shows that we have about 100 million neurons in our gut. There is a real and primal connection between our brain and our gut. We even talk about "gut feelings". There are hundreds of million of neurons connecting the brain to the enteric nervous system. Our brain and gut are connected by both neurons and hormones that constantly provide feedback about how we are feeling internally. The enteric nervous system is so extensive that it can operate as an independent entity without input from our central nervous system, although they are in regular communication. It seems as if one job of our second brain is to work with the trillions of microorganisms residing in the gut.

The environment within the gut dictates which inhabitants thrive. Microbes relying on the mucus layer will struggle in a gut where mucus is exceedingly sparse and thin. Bulk up the mucus, and the mucus-adapted microbes can stage a comeback. The nervous system, through its ability to affect gut transit time and mucus secretion, can help dictate which microbes inhabit the gut. Communication works the other way too. Not only is our brain aware of our gut microbes but these bacteria can influence our perception of the world and alter our behaviour. Healing gut ecology has even been found to help with autism. The gut microbiota influences the body's level of the neurotransmitter serotonin, which regulates feelings of happiness. About 90% of the body's serotonin is in the gut and 50% of our dopamine.

Probiotics and Prebiotics

Bringing in probiotics to promote healthy microorganisms in the gut and prebiotics to feed them is part of looking after the ecology of our gut. Doing this is very beneficial for both our immune systems and our mental and emotional well-being. To expand, probiotics are foods and drinks and supplements that actually introduce friendly microorganisms. Prebiotics are foods that feed these microorganisms, often because they contains substances that are not digestible to us but are to beneficial microorganisms. Examples are yacon root and black beans. Kefir is the most powerful probiotic I know. It introduces beneficial microorganisms and lays down a film in which they can nest. It also takes out unwanted microorganisms. Fermented foods such as yoghurt and cultured vegetables are also probiotic if they are raw and unpasteurised. Colostrum is another probiotic food that can be very helpful for people who react to stronger foods such as kefir.

Be aware of factors that wipe out internal flora for example chlorine in municipal tap water and antibiotics. If you do find yourself using these things you can take probiotics afterwards to restore your internal ecosystem. It's good to include probiotics with every meal if possible, whether you use kefir, fermented vegetables or even probiotic superfood mixes you can purchase. Raw Reserve is my favourite.

Colon Cleansing

Cleansing is a huge topic. In this book I just point you to the areas of cleansing to look into if you are not doing so already. If you have not embarked on this kind of activity before the list looks daunting. It's not worth getting overwhelmed, approach it piece by piece, in due course. Colon and liver cleansing are the priority for most people. A diet predominantly consisting of raw fruit and vegetables will naturally stimulate a cleansing process, but for optimal state of well being and speeding the process along it's definitely worth taking some cleansing steps. Afterwards we feel lighter, we absorb nutrients better and feel more of a natural high eating a natural diet.

In most cases I would say start with the digestive system oxygen cleanse using a product like oxymag. You will begin to remove old waste material and speed up digestion. With this particular product you just mix a spoonful of the powder with water and ingest followed by citrus juice to activate it.

Colonic hydrotherapy (cleaning out the large intestine with water, carried out by a professional colon hydrotherapist) is a great second step. An initial colonic will soften waste material and so it's recommended to have another one a week or two later. Then if you are keen there are full intestinal system cleanses such as the Ejuva which cleanse the entire digestive tract. Hardly any of us have avoided problematic foods during our life times, and this is a chance to get a bit of a fresh start. Eating sprouts such as alfalfa sprouts over a long period tends to maintain a cleaner digestive system and reduce the build up of waste. After colonics it's important to take probiotics to restore the ecosystem of the gut.

Another less intrusive option is the C cleanse. Start on an empty stomach, first thing in the morning. Dissolve a half-teaspoon of high quality buffered vitamin C Buffered Powder (1.5 grams) in water and drink. The amount of C you need depends on how quickly your body uses it up. A healthy person should begin with a level half-teaspoon dissolved in water every 15 minutes. A moderately healthy person should start with 1 teaspoon every 15 minutes. A person in ill health would start with 2 teaspoons every 15 minutes. Continue until you reach a watery stool or an enema-like evacuation of liquid. Do not stop at loose stool. You want to energise the body to flush out toxins and reduce the risk that they may recirculate and induce problems. After this happen, stop consuming the C for the day.

Liver Cleansing

Liver cleansing is a good next step. Over the years debris in the liver and gall bladder are coated by the body as a protective measure and build up to be stones which block the function of both these organs. Malic acid in apple cider vinegar can break these stones down. A dose of olive oil and citrus juice then stimulates the liver and gall bladder and the stones are flushed out. It can be quite a dramatic and exciting event! Some people are equally excited too about the way they feel afterwards and their improved ability to digest fats and food in general. There is a whole protocol described in 'The Amazing Liver and Gallbladder Flush' byAndreas Moritz. In the lead up week, as well as taking apple cider vinegar you can also prepare by eating only blended raw foods and taking an oxygen cleanse so that when the stones are released they pass easily out of the intestines. Afterwards a colonic hydrotherapy session is highly recommended to move stones out of the system.

Kidney Cleansing

Kidney cleansing foods include cranberries, blueberries celery, parley, dandelion root, nettle, and uva ursi. Chanca Piedra, known as the stone breaker is an Amazonian remedy for kidney stones, gall stones and general decalcification and it's worth doing a course of it from time to time. Of course drinking plenty of good clean fresh water is important for the kidneys.

Skin Brushing

Skin brushing using a purpose made skin brush helps the kidneys and is a generally good wake up practice. Although our blood is pumped around our body our lymph fluid needs the stimulation of exercise or brushing. The lymph fluid transports nutrients and removes waste materials to and from deeper in the body tissues than blood. A clean natural bristle shoe brush kept for the purpose works well on the face. When people eat raw and high nutrient food for a period of time the skin tends to get stronger so this kind of brushing feels more comfortable.

Fasting

Fasts of one kind or another give the body a rest from digestion so that it can do essential cleansing and repair work. They can range from water only, to just green juices right up to a combination of juices, smoothies or blended foods. These are known as smoothie fasts or feasts. They reset the body and taste buds and afterwards people notice that they are drawn to more alkalising and healthy foods, have less desire for sweet tastes and they generally feel lighter, happier and more energetic. These blended food feasts/fasts nourish the body whilst freeing the body from expending energy on digestion. This means that cleansing and rejuvenation can both happen. Bringing in oxymag or an equivalent product enhances this type of cleansing. Consuming just blended foods and drinks is a good strategy for having lots clear energy. It's a nice undramatic way of resetting your system.

Fat cell cleanses are deep cleanses to remove toxins or old drug residues lurking deep in tissues. It involves a niacin flush. This means taking a large dose of niacin (B3) which breaks open the fat cells where such matter is stored. This needs to be followed by vigorous exercise to mobilise the particles and then a sauna to expel them through the skin. Afterwards you can replace the fats by eating healthy raw unprocessed fats such as avocado, coconut, olives etc. This cleanse needs to be done according to a safe methods as large doses of niacin and also the released toxins can have a big effect on the body. Dr George Yu is one source and I have listed an interview of his in the references.

Other Cleansing Techniques

Sulphur in the form of MSM, preferably organic, can be taken to combine with toxic metals in the body such as mercury, lead and cadmium and escort them out of the body. The dose is generally 1 teaspoon to 1 tablespoon MSM twice a day, increasing the dose if detoxification symptoms occur.

Saunas are great too for cleansing pores and sweating out of waste, leaving skin soft.

Zeolites I have mentioned for carrying out heavy metals including radioactive ones and pesticides. Natural turpentine including resin enriched cedar oil is a great way of getting rid of internal parasites.

8. Reclaiming and Sustaining your Mind

>...when words were like magic
>the human mind had mysterious powers
>a word spoken by chance might have strange consequences
>it would suddenly come alive
>and what people wanted to happen could happen
>
>Inuit poem

The overarching message that I want to share in this chapter is the necessity of connecting with a benign source of wisdom, an organising principle, beyond and bigger than our own minds. After all, how can we organise our own minds with our own minds? This is the neuroticism of these times. We need discernment in choosing the connection we make. There are many influences in this world. How do we choose what to let influence us? Our feelings are our guidance and our self-correction mechanism. Regaining access to our feelings is a key part of this path. Neuroactive nutrition i.e. food and herbs that nourish the neural system are the biochemical foundation that enables us to heighten our senses to a new level. Connection to the Earth and nature connects us to source. We need to plug our minds into the life force. Eating our natural food stuffs, their living structure gives us a real energetic connection to larger and saner forces. I believe this is a feeling we crave as humans. It's a safe feeling where we don't have to orchestrate our whole worlds, but play our part in a much bigger story than us. As I described when I talked about the benefits of raw foods, undamaged biological material has a fractal structure which facilitates the transmission of information. It also builds, nourishes and activates the neural system. The human story has been shaped by brain biochemicals. Change our neural chemistry and the story changes.

Getting this neurochemistry into place has been the subject of the first part of this book. In this chapter I talk about how you can reclaim our minds from cultural conditioning and the distractions of the information age. Also how you can deal with intrusions into your mind and find sense and wisdom through connecting to the mind of nature and divine intelligence. I talk about how we can work round the split brain situation, the fact that our left hemispheres are retarded and right hemispheres suppressed.

Humans have the ability to experiment and make errors. They are also endowed with a self-correcting feature. The glitch in our development has made this self-monitoring feature more difficult to access. This glitch, the loss of forest biochemistry, the deficient reading of the DNA and the retardation of the left hemisphere is a situation that we are not, so far, equipped to deal with. For example one of the symptoms is confabulation, lying without knowing it. As a result of this the world today is saturated with deception. Yet we are by nature trusting. We need to develop the ability to discern more.

Where we are at in our minds today

The way we use our minds is probably quite recent. Even a few thousand years ago it seems people routinely heard what they described as the voices of the gods inspiring them and took guidance from the signs and omens of nature. This all might sound ridiculous to many people today but then we were at a stage where the right hemisphere was less strangulated and was more accessible. We had a split brain but the hemispheres were more equal so we understood our world in terms of god-like consciousness and human consciousness. I feel that originally, before the split brain, as humans we would have felt ourselves to be part of a bigger life force, and we would have had a whole brain consciousness. This was a long time ago and could happen again. Meanwhile in split brain consciousness, looking at tribes not so long ago, there was provision for initiation into expanded consciousness , there were nurturing and guiding steps in place. In our modern world, there is little guidance at all. Although we have the ancient teachings of the world available to us, by themselves they may make little sense to us because we are in such a different state and situation to when they were written. New knowledge is needed, couched in terms we understand today. We need matter of fact knowledge, practical strategies, that we can implement quickly and get results.

The Split Brain Experience

Because of our split brains we are able to experience feelings and thoughts that are at odds with each other. We are also able to conceal our true intensions behind our actions. We have even developed he ability to act without intention. Or desires and actions have become dislocated. We try to work many things out because we have lost the sense of being guided. Our imaginations become filled with fearful images.

"As natural humans, instinct, simplicity, and sensitivity would also guide us, as through a dance or geometric pattern, the design of which we would intuitively know. This is how primitive people are able to not care about whether they will eat tomorrow. It is this ancient instinct and natural connectivity that is now considered to be irrational and unreliable" says C. G. Browne in her book Forbidden Dimensions.

This natural way of using of the mind in collaboration with divine intelligence, I believe can ultimately be found again.

Dealing with Intrusion into our Natural Thought Processes

Because of what has happened to us there is now a massive amount of misleading information in the world and it is very difficult for us to tell what is true and what isn't. Confabulation, in other words lying without being aware of it is, as we saw in chapter 2, is a fact of life due to the situation of a dominant yet limited left cerebral hemisphere that is not in touch with actual reality. And because of this limitation it is difficult for us to distinguish what is actually true and relevant. Our minds can be pulled here, there and everywhere in a way that if it were happening to our bodies, would obviously ridiculous.

It is taken for granted as a fact of life that most of our mental powers are unconscious but if the glitch in our neural system were healed then who knows? With two fully functioning cerebral hemispheres, or even only one unsuppressed functioning hemisphere, we could have vast awareness and be linked in to the mind of nature, divine intelligence. Even now, through the more intact right hemisphere, we can find connection to natural intelligence, creativity, enhanced imagination, inspiration and intuition, unexpected solutions to problems, and feelings of safety, abundance, variety and connection. Instead of wasting our thoughts complaining about the situation we can allow them to become inspired by the wisdom of source and tune into solutions. We can find a genuine sense of our own purpose and goals. If we put this together with generally good patterns of positive thinking our lives start to take shape. These strategies seem obvious but if we actually do them consistently then life changes. The basic framework is being in natural surroundings or with natural stimuli, naturally neuroactive nutrition, calming the left hemisphere, vitalising the right hemisphere and being aware of the way we use our minds.

Left hemisphere function is retarded and limited. It seems like logic but it is without the checks and balances of outside reality. It's programmed thoughts, which in themselves may seem to make logical sense but have little bearing on what is actually happening. With our senses of feeling and purpose muted it's easy to get carried off on a string of purposeless and possibly painful thought processes.. When we get distracted from this we can get at worst very miserable and at the least less productive than we could be. It's tempting to give these thoughts and ideas more power than they actually have. In reality they come about through our species wide insanity. As Tony Wright explains, this is not a mild condition affecting a few people, this is a serious condition that affects us all. Psychopaths are just the ones who are most damaged.

In the biological model the problem is described as coming from the left hemisphere of the brain. Ancient mythology also has a way of describing the situation. Archons is a term reintroduced into public awareness by Gnostic scholar John Lash and refers to mind parasites, with no intention of their own and unable to physically live in the Earth's atmosphere, which piggy back on human intention. The archons have a particularly strong hold on some groups of humans, and they have become the dominant ones in our world. Sometimes known as intra-species predators (they prey on other humans) or psychopaths, we would be wise not to ascribe them more power than they have. Benign natural and supernatural forces and the life force itself are infinitely more powerful. By giving them power in our minds we actually give them our own power. Power is ideally a power sharing arrangement with the benign and divine forces. Archons can be seen as agents of discord. Random and senseless thoughts are really not worth analysing. If we try to make sense of things that don't make sense we can lose our minds in the process. Unfortunately humans have become more interested in their own minds than the mind of nature which has the knowledge to lift us out of all of this.

To quote John Lash:

"Something extremely weird is happening on Earth due to a fissure in the human mind, and this fissure in turn arises from an anomaly in the cosmic order.

The world system we inhabit came about by a mistake" (The Gospel of Philip, NHC II, 3, 75.1)

The magical journey of awareness in which we co-evolve with Gaia's Dreaming is deviated or distorted by an alien influence, so the Gnostics taught. On this recondite point they seem to have agreed with the Yaqui shaman don Juan, who said to Carlos Castaneda, "Human beings are on a journey of awareness, which has been momentarily interrupted by extraneous forces.

Everything we learn about the Archons teaches us something crucial about ourselves"

Connecting into natural imagination and our feeling-awareness and remaining focused on our goals within that is essential to our sanity. As important is recognising the delusory nature of our stream of fearful, anxious thoughts.
The practical steps in this chapter are designed to help us do this. I have already talked about natural neuroactive nutrition and natural living. Now I'll go through the ways we can calm our left hemispheres and boost our right hemispheres. Then I'll move onto specific ways we can reclaim the use of our thinking processes.

Shifting Hemispheres

Reducing left hemisphere stranglehold and increasing right hemisphere access is both calming and energising. The same is true of natural neuroactive nutrition. The starting point, in our chaotic world, is surely a place of calm. Calm and centred is connected to the fractal web of life, the natural intelligence, through which we can make sense of everything. We are told that in nature it's a fight for survival yet when we go into nature, unless we are entering a natural disaster area it has qualities of harmony. Life flourishes in peaceful surroundings. To do as much as possible in an aware, emotionally sober 'mindful' state is actually more efficient as well as more pleasant and therapeutic. We lose awareness of the passing of time and stop wanting it to slow down or speed up and actually make better use of it. The activities that come from this state of mind are more genuinely productive and integrated into reality and actually take us to where we would like to go faster. It puts us on the right footing for achieving things of lasting value.

Real, strong energy is relaxed because it is harmonious. When our brains are working better we will feel relaxed, we have less to be anxious about because we are more empowered and more in touch with moment by moment energetic reality This is a much safer place to be than out of touch with reality! When we feel energised and connected inside we can become calm because we are not reaching out desperately for energy from others. We are connected to source. In this state we are more sensitive to others feelings. I think most of us experience a range of states, that's one reason why a sense of community and friendship are so important so we can help each other hold a state of calm awareness.

As we calm the left hemisphere the creativity of the right hemisphere starts to blossom. The problems we have created cannot be solved at the level of consciousness that created them. When the conceptual mind thinks 'not' something we are still creating the 'something'. We cannot *not* imagine something! That is what is meant by the unconscious does not understand a negative. That is why positive thinking is so powerful. Actually it is the feeling state (which is so often unconscious) that does not feel a negative – it feels things that are there, not that are not there! As we become more aware of our mental imagery we will automatically choose more imagery that we like. Imagining what we would like consistently - this sounds a clear note in the world of noise.

Summary of techniques that enhance right brain function and/or reduce left brain influence.

We can reduce the dominance of the left hemisphere and have a more right hemisphered experience by doing many things which we have probably already noticed make us feel good. They also make us function better overall and lead more meaningful, purposeful lives. Pleasure cannot be experienced through the left hemisphere, only the right. When we are out of kilter it's a sign we need to remember to do these things. There are a myriad of enjoyable techniques which quieten the left hemisphere and boost right hemisphere activity. Many of the traditional spiritual practices were designed to do just this. We can fruitfully engage in them or the modern equivalents.

As we incorporate these activities and ways of being into our lives, our 'minds' become calmer whilst our powers of creative imagery soar. As our creative minds become more fired up and empowered, ironically, we can actually feel more relaxed. The conceptual left hemisphere needs to rapidly update in the light of new information so that it can work with the right hemisphere's visions of the most desirable futures we can imagine. At the same time we need to remain rooted and able to function authentically in current reality by staying in our body and feeling awareness (right hemisphere function) and not carried off by the new ideas into a world of conceptualisation which is the problem in the first place.

Naturally Neuroactive Diet
- nutrient dense raw food diet with undamaged fatty acids, amino acids and fruit compounds
- appropriate judicious biochemical supplementation, to supply missing neural chemistry, to stimulate right hemisphere and also the pineal gland to pump its own biochemicals.

Quietening the mind
- reducing speaking, thinking and conceptualising, instead thinking in pictures
- meditative activities, yoga, relaxation, carrying out daily activities in a meditative state, staying in body, visual and sensual awareness.

Gentle Techniques
- daydreaming/fantasising/use of imagination, visions of the future
- staring
- looking up e.g. at the sky or stars, flying kites, mountain climbing
- music, preferably complex flowing music
- dancing or rather allowing ones body to move with music
- being in nature, energetic places, star watching, listening to bird song
- sensory experiences – art, colour, use of incense etc.
- creative and artistic pursuits
- loving touch
- using left hand
- laughter and humour
- using a neurophone (Patrick Flanagan's invention)
- earthing
- yoga

Powerful Techniques
- plant medicines
- stimulation of pineal
- sleep deprivation - 'staying awake' for one or more nights/reducing sleep at a comfortable level
- eye connection/mirror gazing

While sleep deprivation is a very powerful tool for experiencing expanded states of consciousness, *in our current state* it cannot be maintained indefinitely. We need more extended periods of sleep at times to maintain our bodies and health; when we sleep we go into deep states of consciousness, currently quite difficult for most of us to access while awake, where biochemical changes facilitate healing and growth.

The combination of raw naturally neuroactive food, plant medicines and sleep deprivation are the most powerful shamanic tools known.

Tantra or sacred sex is an attempt to rediscover right hemisphere or whole brain sex. Psychoactive substances and sex are our two remaining most accessible doorways to that state of consciousness we long to be in. Unfortunately our hormonal and neurological imbalances have distorted the experience. Tantric methods of one kind or another are an attempt to bring sex to the connected level we sense it could be. Sexual interaction bathed in the combination of not only our sex hormones but ample plant chemistry through natural nutrition and reestablished pineal chemistry would take us to another dimension of experience, one known of old.

Humour jettisons us out of limited left brain perspective by various means such as putting two incongruent things together, moving something into a very different context or simply describing things as they are when they are ridiculous. It sounds very clinical, but smiling and laughter are actually signs of shifting hemispheres, from left to right. Humour breaks the left hemisphere spell. At the end of a laugh we are free. When you begin to see the situation we are in as humans there is plenty to laugh about. It really is very ludicrous and there are plenty of opportunities for the benefits of humour to come in. When we are already engrossed in a very right hemisphere pursuit it may seem irrelevant because we are already there. The unconscious does not have a sense of humour and so cynical humour soon outgrows its usefulness on this path as our mood lifts!

Vipassanā style meditation. Vipassanā means to see things as they really are. It is one of the most ancient techniques of meditation and involves body awareness and watching the mind. Doing this brings us back into actual energetic reality and reduces our tendency to be disturbed by our thoughts.

We can weave these ways of being into our lives and they become habitual. We get into the practice of making ourselves feel good, at nurturing our brains in this way.

Mental Habits

As we become lucid enough to see how much creative input we have into our life experiences and start to make more informed choices regarding our thoughts and actions our lives can become significantly better. It becomes obvious on a moment by moment level that life is indeed a precious gift and not the burden that we have at times experienced it as! The very fact that we have choices makes it a gift rather than a burden. The trick is really not to get caught up in physical circumstances rather take a mental step back and think about how we would like life to be, and work from there, weaving this into what we currently have on our plates. There are many unhelpful things we have been told but perhaps the most insidious one is that it is somehow virtuous to suffer and it is through doing so that we will deserve reward. Actually nothing could be further from the truth and if the most significant spiritual truth is that we are all connected then surely the best thing we can all do for ourselves and each other is feel better.

In addition to the physical things we can do to make ourselves better there are some mental habits we can adopt that can transform the quality of our lives. I'll list some very straightforward ones here then go deeper into the qualities that make us human.

Gratitude

Soon after waking if we can think of a few things or at least one thing we are truly grateful for it starts the ball rolling for the day. When we focus on gratitude it tends to attract more things into our lives that make us feel there way we want to. The reason for practising gratitude is not just that we have so much to be grateful for. The second reason is that gratitude itself makes us feel better. Choosing to think about what is desirable to us rather than what we don't want is a related practice.

Positive Thinking

Question your beliefs and whether they are they true because they impact how you feel.

Years ago I made a resolution that I was going to think 100% positive. Great idea. Then I wondered, what am I going to think about. It reminded me of a resolution I had made years before to eat my food 100% raw. The next question was what am I actually going to eat? It took some thinking through and I did find a way that worked for me long term. Eventually it did include some cooked foods and drinks that I find beneficial more than problematic but it is predominantly raw food. In that way I feel better than even 100%. With thinking I feel it's the same. Predominantly positive thinking with a sense of gratitude for what already exists, goals for what we would like and some room to think about matters that we want to think about. The main thing as I always emphasise it to be aware of the impact of our thoughts.

Spending all our time remarking how wonderful life is and saying that everything is good is of course not authentic or the complete picture and not necessary. We have stuff to do and it is also authentic to acknowledge thats sometimes we don't feel great and there are matters to be resolved. There is generally a positive uplifting way to do it though.

There is a trick to the mental suggestions we give ourselves and others - and the truth is everything we think and say is a suggestion. If you want to give yourself powerful suggestions then keep them in the present, specific, succinct, positive and with feeling and imagery. Repeat them then let them go out of your conscious (left hemisphere dominated) mind. One technique is to create a special place in the mind where nothing and nobody can worry or disturb us. Here we can create what we would like, the images and feelings that nourish and inspire us – and revisit when we need rejuvenation - the place of our dreams. Ideally this paradisiacal place would start to expand into our lives.

The past can be seen as a place in our minds where we store a treasure-house of memories – images and resources we can draw on. The future is a place in our minds of endless possibilities where we an create our visions and dreams. The present moment is the place we can act in, create practically, decide our moment by moment course of action, and achieve, nourished and assisted by those memories and dreams in whatever way we choose. We are in the creative moment right now. The present moment is the only place anything physical can be done – fortunately it will go on forever – and we feel a lot better immediately we think and act positively within it.

Managing our thoughts and energetic state is something that most of us neglect until they make life so painful that we have to reconsider. We need to bear in mind that our limited conceptual thoughts are left hemisphere function and we are stuck with them for the moment even if we manage to reduce their volume, velocity and intensity by calming the left hemisphere and boosting the right. We can learn to deal with them much more effectively. The first step is to be aware of them. This is much easier when we have optimal brain chemistry in place and are actively shifting towards the right hemisphere, because it is the right hemisphere with optimal biochemistry that has awareness. Language is one of the areas most dominated by the left hemisphere and thoughts are from a limited perspective and not necessarily true. We do not need to define ourselves by them. The ultimate meaning of life is not an intellectual answer - it is a way of being. And whilst talking has its place it does not ultimately get us there. As we begin to boost the right hemisphere more, we get clearer intuitions and begin to be be able to follow where our energy is going rather than our thoughts. We have more energy for our tasks this way. And by simple awareness of how we feel, the thoughts and images in our heads, the energies in our bodies, the energetic signals from those around us and our environment, we will naturally choose more helpful and uplifting mental images and thought patterns and behaviours.

Accurate thinking is not just about asking whether something is actually true but whether it is relevant to where we want go, what we are aiming at.

A trap to avoid is the quest for perfection. It's not really a human quality and trying to achieve it stifles creativity and wastes life. As someone put it to me, 20% of the time spent on a task will be getting it right, then the next 80% trying to make it perfect and making it worse.

Routines and Rituals

It's said that successful people don't rely on willpower they rely on rituals. It takes you a few weeks to install desirable habits, after that they are hard to break. After about 21 days they become easy. After about 65 days they are entrenched and it's hard not to do them. They can give you trust in yourself and free you to get on with what you want to do. Installing an early morning routine of connection to nature, exercise, journalling, sacred rituals, study, and dealing with emails frees up the rest of the day to plunge into projects that are really going to make a difference or activities we really enjoy. The transition between sleeping and waking is one of the most difficult parts of the day to manage. When we are asleep the left hemisphere is quietened and right hemisphere activity takes over. After sleeping the left hemisphere is refreshed and reinstates its dominance with all it's limitations and fears. It's like going through a mini fall from grace each day. This is why waking rituals are so helpful to make this transition into the activity of the day. It's easy to neglect our key life projects attending to small easy tasks, or let the apparent urgency of small tasks tale us away from the parts of our lives we really love. It's so important to make time for the big projects that will really make a difference in our lives and work. They should be prioritised straight after the immediate things that need doing each day.

Reducing Complaining

Sometimes complaining can make people feel more miserable than the thing they are actually complaining about. The reason to minimise complaining is not that we have nothing to complain about, but that it makes us, and whoever is on the receiving end feel terrible. This is so different to bringing up problems that need solutions. It's different in its intent. The difference is between focusing on the problem and focusing on the solution. The thing to be aware of is that the words we use create images in our minds.

Complaining causes us and those around us additional distress and has an emotional component that tends to keep us locked into problems. Sometimes we do not have control of circumstances but we do have control of how we respond to them. People often do not realise what a destructive force habitual complaining has been in their lives until they stop doing it. Complaining changes the wiring of our brains. (see the article *Complaining is Terrible for you according to Science* by Jessica Stillman). Gratitude is a great antidote. Complaining is very contagious because before we know it we can find ourselves complaining about people complaining ! It's a symptom of the emotional plague described by Wilhelm Reich.

Dealing with Emotions

Allowing ourselves to experience the full range full range of emotions with enthusiasm brings us into a state of enthusiasm for life. That does not mean necessarily expressing them out in the world, rather experiencing them fully. We cannot cure judgement of other people with judgement. Enthusiastically feeling our emotions gets us back into that feeling of enthusiasm for life. One of the greatest pains we can experience is to not be fully living our a true sense of purpose and destiny. Commitment to this can get us through a lot.

Thought Field Therapy or Emotional Freedom Techniques, TFT or EFT as it is more commonly known is recognised as one of the most powerful tools in the field of energy medicine and transformation. It is a blend of Chinese medicine and modern psychology in which you take two fingers and tap on specific parts of the body that are located on what Chinese medicine calls meridians. According to Chinese medicine these pathways often become blocked which leads to problems in the physical organism. Traditionally Chinese medicine uses various techniques to rectify these blockages most notably acupuncture. Roger Callaghan discovered this technique basically by accident during the earlier part of his career as a psychologist. He was working with one of his clients who had severe phobia of water to the point where she couldn't even give her children baths. One day he asked her where exactly on the body was the source of her emotional distress. She replied "in my gut around the solar plexus area". He had just come back from Asia where he had been studying rudimentary Chinese medicine and he remembered that the point on the bone below the eye corresponds to to that part of the body. He got a hunch and told her to tap the point while thinking about her phobia. She did as he instructed and, to cut along story short, her phobia was gone permanently.

He later went on to experiment with other acupuncture points and various sequences of tapping and came up with the modality called

Thought Field Therapy. One of his students, Gary Craig later came up with emotional freedom technique or EFT which is just a slight variation but is basically just as effective. This kind of technique can seem kind of strange and is easy to miss or disregard, but it is one of the most powerful and effective ways to change your emotional state and can even transform long standing core beliefs. It is very easy to learn and can be applied in a few minutes on most issues. . You can download a free guide to tapping at Roger Callahan's site, www.rogercallahan.com and www.thetappingsolution.com and a free guide to EFT at Gary Craig's site www.garythink.com.

The tapping routine is very quick, simple and straightforward. Times when we are emotionally uncomfortable become ideal opportunities to permanently clear long-standing issues and access resources within ourselves that we never realised we had. Discord with or the loss of another person from our lives is the hardest pain that most of us experience. There is a tailored tapping routine that can relieve this kind of trauma that might otherwise take months or even years of grieving. Grieving is important to go through thoroughly when we experience loss of a loved one, so that we can continue to be fully here. In current times when so much is falling away to make way for the new, the ability to grieve is more crucial than ever.

A Sense of Purpose

This may even be the starting point of it all and the main key to fulfilment. It is a way of channelling our desires in a constructive way that benefits ourselves and others long term. It can begin as a simple desire to feel good and to discover our life purpose. Our goals connect us to our purpose in life. They need to be big enough to excite us and manageable enough so that we know we can achieve them. Then we feel good thinking about them and working toward them, thus enabling us to delay some gratification in order to experience greater reward in the future. This practice in itself significantly increases our sense of well-being and keeps levels of dopamine, the enthusiasm neurotransmitter, high. The wonderful thing about purpose is that we can have one whatever circumstances we find ourselves in. In some ways our sense of purpose and aim defines who we are more than anything else. Living our purpose connects us with the life force and gives us energy we would not otherwise have.

A Commitment to Turn all Circumstances to Advantage

When things fail to go according to plan or 'go wrong' we decide that we will create something beneficial out of whatever has happened. Not only does this create great benefits for us in our lives but it also gives us an inner confidence that no matter what happens, we can deal with it and things will ultimately turn out well. This attitude in itself can bring miracles into our lives.

As we put these methods into practice not only does life become more enjoyable and productive, the way forward to more solutions becomes clear. The next steps reveal themselves. Consistency and momentum are key. Of course there will be setbacks but the important thing is the wholehearted commitment to keep moving forward. We need to stay focused in solution mode, whilst being aware of the problems.

Cultivating Human Mental Characteristics

When we think about the way we use our minds we need to be aware of what they are designed to do. You could correlate these in some way to Abraham Maslow's hierarchy of needs, to the chakras and endocrine system and so forth. Our characteristics do correlate with biochemicals. This list comes from the Gnostic research of John Lash and I have added my own observations.

Connection to Divine Intelligence

Called nous by the Gnostics this is our natural intelligence and ability to feel. It is the awareness experienced by all living things. In order to experience it we need to plug our minds back into the life force.

We need to plug our minds back into the life force.

In the words of Gnostic scholar John Lash "The human species receives from the intelligence of the Earth a special dose of self-corrective savvy (sapience). The wisdom endowment (as it may be called) is the source of our instinctual capacities as well as our ethical sense. This precious endowment, called nous by Gnostics, must be cultivated in order for us to realize it. Failing to cultivate it, we risk becoming something less than human. Unlike other species, who are more closely bound to their instinctual patterns, we have huge latitude to wander and err, but this also allows us to explore, invent, imagine. We learn by making errors and correcting them, thanks to the self-correcting element in nous, our self-monitoring noetic faculty."

Language

Dianoia is a beautiful word that describes our capacity for communication and language.

Tony Wright, describes speech as a singing impediment. This sounds right to me. The left hemisphere has simply lost the ability to be musical in its communications. Singing is a language experience and also a feeling experience. It's more than a conveyance of concepts which represent what we are are describing. Poetry and poetic speech are similar in this way. I feel that original singing would be something like a human sophisticated version of birdsong rather than the stylised music of today or in the words of Richard Leviton in '*Voices from the Dreamtime, The Aboriginal*

*Vision and Wester Culture'"*creative mantric sound". The songs and music of nature are complex vibrational patterns which we potentially have the ability to tune into just as the Aborigines did.

"The plants and trees sing to us humans silently, and all they ask in return is for us to sing to them."Marlo Morgan in *Mutant Message Down Under.*

Stories and Patterns

Humans live by stories. In any case the narrative is important and if we don't choose a narrative to live by then we fall into the default one of the collective. Being able to see patterns and create new models is also one of our abilities. DMT is the essential neurotransmitter that helps us do this. Our sense of being self-directing and our need to live a life story that means something to us is, I think, why 85% of people feel they have a book to write. We need a grand narrative to place our individual stories in, just as we need our homes to be placed in a larger setting. Dreaming our story embedded to the bigger story of humanity and the planet is an integral part of being human. The earth is the wholesome source, setting and story behind our stories. We need to take care not to get too embroiled in the stories of the human predators, the psychopaths in our society, who know only power but not empathy. They - like monsters in fairy tales, are only part of the story. If we are more designed to sing or talk in a sing song manner, then maybe our narratives could be viewed as more like a musical, set within the song of nature.

Perinoia or Playfulness

Perinoia is our ability to pretend, to make things up (in a good way), our capacity for novelty. It's our spontaneous playfulness.

Robert Lawlor describes the culture of one tribe of aborigines whose culture was not dominated by survival strategies. By the time an individual was five they could take care of their own modest survival needs with a small percentage of their time. Socialising was something then done for the sheer pleasure of it rather than to carry out commercial transactions. Walking and dancing were key activities. In the words of Robert Lawlor "the principle of the culture is simply walking ... moving through a free open space and enjoying the mystery and beauty of a world that is undisturbed by the presence of any form of life ... what the neuromuscular movement of walking actually does round the spinal column is to set up an imploding vortex of bioenergetic field and it's not while standing still it's only when walking so walking and dancing are the fundamental ground of aboriginal culture not the struggle to provide the subsidence and basis of life and that's a major psychological and psycho spiritual shift in the orientation between agriculture and hunting and gathering".

Humans' ability to make things up in the context of the ongoing anxiety that we experience as a result of left hemisphere damage can cause paranoia.

Desire, Passion and Enthusiasm

Known as enthymesis, this is part of being human. As one desire gets satisfied, another one arises. This is inherent in being human. Desire is the feeling of the life force. Although the Buddha taught to the world at large that desire or attachment is the cause of all suffering, to his inner circle he taught liberation through the fulfilment of desire. Desires are not necessarily selfish, they can include the desire to love and grow for example and they can be transpersonal. When we attune to our true natural desires, we may find that what we desire is already coming towards us, it is destined for us, it is just for us to move towards it. True natural desires are gifts from the divine. They are guiding us to where we are meant to be going.

In general it's good to be focused on what we desire and on generally desirable outcomes for all. It's surprising how much time we all waste focused on undesirable outcomes not realising how much we add to them. One of the most important tasks is to identify our highest desire. We need to keep our focus on things that are believable to us. Although it's good to set time goals for our own tasks, when it comes to our wishes coming true it's wise to leave the timing open so we don't get disillusioned. The expansion of awareness obtained by following the steps to engage and nourish our right hemispheres obviously helps too. Knowing that we are moving towards what we want makes it real in our imagination and then we are half way there.

It's so important to know what we want. If we don't we default into victim consciousness. To know our deepest desire, and stick with it is a high commitment to make. We are surrendered to whether we attain it or not, and open to its fulfilment in ways we cannot predict or even understand.

Free Will and Intention

Known as ennoia, humans have free will. We have freedom form instinctual programs and can set our intentions. We are designed to have the ability to self-correct when we make errors. We are teleological i.e. we feel our best when working towards goals, our desires. We are designed to have a sense of direction and of destiny. Goal focus is that sense of direction which enables us to enjoy the present moment. Freedom is little use to us without a sense of purpose.

Freedom is little use without a sense of purpose.

Dopamine levels remain high while we are working towards a goal, dropping when we achieve it. By engaging with the next goal we get our dopamine levels up again. Making effort to get what we desire is an essential part of well-being. Dopamine levels are kept high by delayed gratification and they drop when we get what we want. We move endlessly through these desires and when they are healthy and achievable there is no reason to let this worry us.

Wisdom

As humans we have genius learning abilities and intense curiosity. True wisdom comes through connection with nature and the reality of life and the ability to connect to the planetary mind.

Creative Imagination

Our capacity for free will, our ability to pretend and to build abstract models, gives us the capacity to disconnect from our environment, which can be a problem. Creative imagination gives us the capacity to solve the problems we have caused for ourselves. We need to distinguish between human and divine imagination. Restoration of human imagination is an essential part of the correction on this planet.

Magic and the Supernatural

The supernatural is simply the realms of nature that are beyond our ordinary everyday awareness. It has only become strange to modern humans because of the shut down in awareness, so it seems other worldly. Because of our lessened ability to connect with the supernatural there are many fraudulent claims which make it even more open to scepticism. The supernatural is what is behind the natural. There would be no natural phenomena if there was no supernatural.

Magic is the human activity of making things with imagination and intention through the powers of the unconscious mind and supernatural. These are abilities beyond the linear logical parts of the mind. It's innate to us. It has become subject of superstition simply because we have lost touch with many of our innate abilities and senses. Sympathetic magic is one of the oldest forms. It's a way of accessing powers within ourselves that we are not always conscious of and bypassing the limitations of the left hemisphere. The so-called 'law of attraction' making of dream boards and so forth to form strong clear consistent images in our minds works along similar principles. People tend to get just what they imagine rather than the conceptual version - and in ways they could not work our logically. That's the power of working around the left hemisphere. When we nourish our neural systems and boost our right hemispheres this process is way more powerful and effective for obvious reasons. Without consciously putting things in place to bring about results we desire, we easily fall into victim consciousness. Indigenous people were often obliged to disguise their magical workings in the face of outside conquest. In Ireland, Haiti and Central America for example, old magic was disguised within a facade of Christian worship. The old ways were gradually forgotten by many. We forgot how to work with our own subconscious and supernatural forces in an act of co-creation. Writing your goals and visions in blue ink on white paper is a simple and clearly sane example of magical working.

There are ten dimensions to existence although only seven of them concern our human existence. You can get a feel for them in this demonstration put together by Rob Bryanton at this site tenthdimension.com. It may be more accurate to substitute galaxy where he says universe, but in any case you get the idea. The first three are the three dimensional reality of space. The fourth is duration or time. We are routinely aware of these four dimensions.

The fifth concerns our choices, or chance in physical reality. This is where our creativity comes in, which involved choices and decisions. Our creativity is impaired by the neurological condition we are in as a species and it's something people notice an improvement in when they put into place nutritional and lifestyle changes. Without our creativity we find ourselves in victim mode.

The sixth dimension comes in when we move between events in a way that in so-called ordinary consciousness we would not think possible. It is the realm of our imaginations, of the dream life we encounter when sleeping or when daydreaming. It seems like we can move to events that to our logical minds would only be possible if the past, or our perception of the past, changed. We can develop the ability to hold a vision of the timeline we want to move to, and act from that, even though at first the sensory input seems at odds with it. In the seventh dimension we encounter all possibilities in our lives, we can connect with our true destiny. This is accessed through the mirroring attention, it's the feeling of being seen by our source, the electrical being that is the earth and dreaming us. I will come back to this in a sequel to this book. It can reach a point where it feels like you have a dowser in the top of the head, I feel sure this is our natural state.

There are some simple steps to changing our life timelines in a way that is beyond our logical understanding. First you visualise what you want to happen. Then you imagine the feeling state that puts you in, hold it and act from that state. Persevere, for a while you are imagining one situation while observing a different one, you are living in two worlds simultaneously. The ability to do this is something we all have and do as part of our lives. We can consciously make it more powerful.

"All creatures, organic and inorganic, human and non-human, live and die by the Dreamings that play through them. In the Aboriginal worldview the unique gift of humans to create culture stems from our capacity to remember and retell the Dreaming, not only of our own species, but of others as well. The indigenous belief that the role of humanity is to remember the events of the Dreaming for all creatures accords with the suggestion presented in *'Sharing the Gaia Mythos: the human species enables a memory-circuit for Gaia.'* by John Lash.

The social sphere is very much constructed around language which has become dominated by the left hemisphere, so it has become necessary for humans to be silent or at least non verbal and retreat from normal society to access this expanded awareness. Social life and the time to be connected to source often have to be separated for this reason. This situation is because of the split brain. When people adjust their brain state, calm the left hemisphere and boost the right it becomes increasingly possible to be in company of each other and at the same time feel connected to source.

The traditional silence of the mysteries has a lot to do with not being able to describe these matters in left brain language without being misunderstood. Experience more than explanations is what is going to transform our lives. That's why I focus on practicalities. That's why I feel practical advice with a rational explanation is needed. What you experience when you change your brain state is something to be discovered when you are there and speculation means very little.

From Victimage to Life Force and Destiny

As we put these methods into practice not only does life become more meaningful, enjoyable and productive, the way forward and the next steps reveal themselves. Consistency and putting all the methods together is what is needed to make it holistic and wholesome. Becoming more sensitive can be uncomfortable as we notice things we had not noticed before. But this gives us the opportunity to change for the better. An awareness of the limited function of our dominant left hemisphere can help us make allowances for others and ourselves. It also helps us understand the structures in our societies and institutions which we have developed to cope, that would be unnecessary for humans in a more attuned state. Things begin to make sense. We can now focus on things that will address the actual cause of the situation. Discovering our highest desire and committing to it, we can play our part in the solution and correction.

The life force is truly stronger than the force of suffering.

Edenic Culture

Culture is the connection between humans and nature, it is about the way we nourish ourselves at every level. Healthy, vibrant and varied cultures arise where humans meet the natural world in their natural state of consciousness. In the loss of our natural state, culture becomes fossilised, but as we regain it, new and novel culture arises spontaneously.

Work, as we move towards this state is something you do that you love and is of value for others and then you are rewarded with something that is of value to you. It is also what we do to get us back to the state we want to be in. Our real physical survival needs are provided for by the planet we live on, and it is possible for humans to have ample amounts of time to spend in activities other than those for survival. Unfortunately money can easily be seen as a way to get everything we want but this as a serious deception.

Although cultures of the past can inspire us regarding what we are capable of, what really excites me is not the idea of going back to the past, but what we are capable of in the future.

If logic tells us that the point of being here is to find a sense of enjoyment and fulfilment in as many moments as then Edenic Culture is focused on this. There is currently a battle for our minds. Our responses to the challenges that face us can be positive, productive playful, humourous and more. If the point is to get into a good state of mind then there is little point in using the problems to justify a problematic state of mind.The art is to stay in the solution not the problem. The task of healing is to clear emotional, electrical and physical blockages so we can fully experience connection to the life force again and the bigger forces than ourselves that orchestrate our lives.

9. Our Hormonal Human Life Cycle

To some extent our individual life cycles are a microcosm of the human story itself. We are conceived into an anomalous situation. From the very start, although our DNA holds the potential for everything we could want or dream of, by the time the cells begin to divide they do so in a biochemical environment in the uterus that is distorted from its original blueprint. Reminiscent of the idea of original sin but not quite the same, it is this biochemical mix that means that we are born with a cerebral left hemisphere that is limited yet dominant, a pineal gland that does not secrete the full quota of its biochemical messengers and a digestive system, immune system and reproductive system that is substantially altered from what it might have been. Here we go through the human life journey, and talk about how this situation is relevant at each stage and also how future generations might be born differently.

I am going to start in terms of the context for the growing up and the sexual differentiation process because it throws so much light on things. I am going to expand on how we can create the best situation possible in growing children's lives, also how we can help with the adult hormonal situation and the gender rift. And then explore how this glitch could be reversed generation by generation.

We can get a sense of the power of hormones when we think about bees. A worker bee is transformed into a queen by the increased ingestion of royal jelly. To quote Tony Wright "The epigenetic effect of royal jelly on a worker bee during the development of a single generation is quite astounding. If a chemical cocktail with the ability to effectively re-interpret the way the DNA code is read were present 24/7 during the evolution of an organism the results would be equally spectacular. A complete re-design and re-engineering at a molecular and cellular level through to a major re-organisation of development, form and function." The changes that happen at adolescence and puberty also show how powerful hormones are; the same DNA is read differently in a different hormonal environment and we go from being boys and girls to men and women.

Puberty

At adolescence we begin to move out of our child like state of innocence into an adult state of consciousness. At this time there is a large drop in melatonin levels which deeply impacts how we feel in ourselves and how we connect to our environment. It changes the way our minds work and our sense of self. This drop in melatonin mirrors what has happened to the human species itself over time with the loss of connection to our own feelings and nature. Also at this time of course the distance between the sexes widens.

If you think about someone in late adolescence they are pretty competent and independent, yet they are not ageing. The neural system is actually still growing until at least the fifties (I suspect beyond); bizarrely we are degenerating before we are even fully developed. The strong suspicion based on what we now know is that we are designed to live way longer than we do now. I will come back to the subject of longevity later in this chapter.

Adolescence and puberty are a tumultuous time because of the profound biochemical changes which change our perceptual state. The adaptations that teenagers go through are adaptations to this change. At this time we need to develop the strategies to handle this new adult chemical state. The left hemisphere increases its dominance even further. With the loss of pineal hormones of course the sex hormones also become more dominant.

Brain development slows down when the melatonin levels drop at this stage. This is one reason why the fall in the average age of puberty over the last century and probably before that is of such cause for concern. It's possible that it is speeded up further by the lowering of melatonin levels by today's levels of electromagnetic radiation. It is also possible it could be delayed by melatonin supplementation but this is something that needs further research.

Sexual Relationships

The premise that we are designed to live in a mixture of not only our own hormones but forest biochemistry tallies with ancient mythology including the sacred connection between man, woman and the Earth. The connection is between male and female and plant hormones. With shared plant chemistry men and women had more in common chemically. Foetal development of males shows us that males are not much more than hormonal variants of females, males and females are genetically almost identical.

Sex itself could be potentially different with a restoration in consciousness. In the words of Tony Wright "If we can recreate our ancestral hormonal environment through diet and a sustained reversal of cerebral dominance, a very different human may emerge. We would experience more profound and pleasurable sexuality too, coupled with a reproductive system that worked as nature intended."
He goes on "We are addicted to sex but could part of this be an addiction to the feeling we get from being momentarily free from our ego-based, fear-ridden, left hemisphere sense of self. Is the sexual drive, which has reached obsessive levels in our society today, a result of a striving to regain something that in our deepest being we know we have lost? At some fundamental level we know there is something more to the sexual experience but, because we don't know where to look, the desire becomes attached to the whole raft of sexual expression from glossy car adverts to the darkest depravity. This distortion arises from a human mind system that has become disconnected from the true needs of the body and from a

more balanced, intuitive and complete side of us. The sexual obsession, which is everywhere in western society (sex sells everything), compensates for the very inefficient reproductive mechanism we are left with today. In fact it has over compensated by a very large factor. We are well out of balance – 7,000,000,000 sex-obsessed humans to date and still copulating!

Melatonin has been used, in trials at least, as the basic ingredient of a contraceptive pill that has been found to stop (what is regarded as) the normal female cycle. This stalled cycle would have been the norm before our ancestors left the forest. Higher melatonin levels resulting from a highly boosted pineal pump would have produced a system that remained in stasis between copulation-induced ovulation/pregnancy events. Hormones are extremely complicated, perplexing and powerful chemicals. There is much more waiting to be discovered about their roles and particularly how they interact with one another. We have seen that as a result of steroid suppression libido calms down but there is evidence that more melatonin can make sex a more pleasurable experience too. Melatonin heightens the effect of our internal endorphins. These are substances that alleviate stress and help to produce sensations of pleasure and relaxed well being. It has even been reported that melatonin, via its stimulation of oxytocin and prolactin, may encourage the physical contact and intimacy that leads to sensual activity. When these hormones were experimentally injected into mice, a dramatic increase in the mouse equivalent of cuddling and hugging took place. Furthermore, when melatonin was added to the evening drinking water of old mice, it was found that not only did they show signs of rejuvenation and increased longevity but also that they engaged in sexual activity again."

On the note of contraception, the research has been released to the public because it was of no commercial use. It was combining large doses of melatonin with small amounts of progesterone and apparently the women trying this found that they felt good on it.

Tony Wright speculates that the primary role of orgasm in the female would have originally been to ovulate, as well as provide pleasure. There is now evidence coming out to support this. "As testosterone is a primary factor in libido (for both sexes), we can speculate that with testosterone modulated by plant hormones, male libido would also be of a different order and it would have been more difficult to reach orgasm ... a sustained amount of sexual activity would have been needed in both males and females to achieve both orgasm and a release of sperm and ova.

Because of our sense of something being missing in our current condition it's very tempting to look for it in another person. This is the basis of co-dependency. Also preoccupation with sex can distract us from experiencing the full spectrum of human experience and life. Putting into place the plant and pineal biochemistry and also connection with the larger energy of nature can help shift this imbalance.

Tantric sex is generally an attempt to make sex more like the way it would be with restored or original consciousness. Or to use sex as a way of improving our state in that direction.

In Marnia Robinson's book 'Cupids Poison Arrow' she describes the problem of our sexual practices in our current state - in particular what happens at orgasm. She points out how dopamine levels crash with orgasm and set up an addictive cycle. She promotes a non-genital orgasm style of sex which increases oxytocin levels and pair-bonding. Sex is a very right hemisphere activity which is wonderful; afterwards there can a rapid return to greater left brain dominance. There is a wealth of evidence that humans can still access prolonged transpersonal states of bliss through sexual union. Even eye connection produces profound shifts. It's just finding the right way of going about it. The connection to and immersion in nature and the bioelectromagnetic aura of the Earth is the key.

When it comes to those psychological differences between men and women, again the things we do for our own well-being also have a positive impact. In particular melatonin increases harmony.

John Gray's observations on the different behaviours of men and women based on their need to boost their own hormone levels are very useful in creating understanding and harmony between the sexes in the times we are in. Even though our sex hormones are problematically dominant due to missing plant and pineal biochemistry, we still have a need to keep them at healthily high levels. Women's habits of spending hours chatting or regularly acting out of unconditional love, for example, boost oxytocin levels which they need to feel right in themselves. A mans' playing competitive sports, hanging out with his male friends or resting before he does a task is boosting his testosterone levels. John Gray expands on this in his book 'Venus on Fire, Mars on Ice: Hormonal Balance--The Key to Life, Love, and Energy'.

What we think of as normal masculinity and femininity is not really optimal. It's interesting to think of all the variations in the ways people experience their sexuality and gender from that perspective.

One of the wonderful things about close one to one relationships is the power of dreaming together. As individuals we have two eyes which gives us a sense of perspective but only one pineal or inner eye. When the two connect we have greater power to manifest.

Babies and Children

When it comes to conceiving children, there is lots of research to be done on how the hormonal environment in utero could be positively and safely changed so that the DNA can be read to produce a child with something nearer optimal potential. It may be that the solution is along the lines of dense natural nutrition plus calming the left hemisphere for the mother. Meanwhile the more nurtured the expectant mother is and the less stress she experiences the better.

Comparing with the life cycles of other mammals it makes sense for a human child to receive their mother's milk to the age of between seven and nine. This mays shock many people but in those later years the child is clearly not feeding like a baby but benefits from various immune and other factors in the mother's milk.

Feeding children high quality nutritionally dense raw food gives them the best start possible, building their neural systems optimally and giving them the opportunity to know what it feels like to feel harmonious within themselves. What's more, the level of contentment, the energy and lovingness of children in this biochemical brain state turns parenting into great joy and fulfilment. The basis is the list for food types I gave in chapter 4. They need greater amounts of some nutrients than adults - for example fat soluble nutrients and it is wise to give raw dairy products to children. It is important that they get a good range of fatty acids including EPA and DHA. Restrictive diets should not be placed on children, rather an abundance of wholesome food. Creating as natural environment as possible and allowing them to enjoy the greater freedom of the right hemisphere which they have when they are young, actually improves their chances for educational progress and achievement later. Waiting until age seven to begin formal instruction in reading and writing is an example of this. The last thing we want to do is hasten the increase in left hemisphere domination. Television, videos and computer activity are best avoided or at least minimised for young children for many reasons, two of which are that they reduce melatonin levels and also they reduce the ability to be self-directed.

To have the privilege of being with people who are not culturally conditioned is an amazing opportunity, you could describe it as an anthropologist's dream. It's a symptom of the topsy-turviness of our world that we have relegated child rearing and childhood itself to the sidelines and children are expected to adapt to the culture rather than the culture being inspired by the expression of more natural humanity displayed by young children. Children's happiness and wellbeing are paramount and our culture really needs to reflect this realisation. Meeting children's needs connects us to our deepest feelings and our potential as humans. Discovering what children's needs are is in many ways discovering human needs.

I had felt there was something very wrong with humans from an early age. When I had my first child, from the moment I looked at him I realised what we humans are is very different to what we have been told. I saw that we have become programmed to be something we are not. I wondered what to do. At this time I was introduced to the 'Continuum Concept' by Jean Liedloff. This was the start of my discovery of natural human lifestyle. Jena Liedloff's work is based on her observations of the Yequana people in Venezuela. She attributed their contentedness to the way they they raised their children.

She emphasised the importance of physical connection in the early years including prolonged breastfeeding, bed-sharing and babies being carried around continuously until they can move by themselves. At the same time it is important that parents have productive purposeful happy lives of their own. Children are welcomed and included but the children are not made the ongoing centre of attention. Adults are available when needed.

She pointed out that a child has tremendous innate sociability and a desire to please and meet the adults expectations. It is helpful to ask children to do the things we want them to do rather than what we don't want them to do.

A young child has an innate understanding of natural dangers – it is the unnatural ones we need to particularly protect them from.

It is confusing for children to be presented with endless choices about things they don't understand. As soon as they show themselves ready and willing it is important that they allowed to make their own decisions in increasing areas of their lives. Firm boundaries work better with young children than endless reasoning.

It is vitally important that children have time and opportunity for creative and make believe games. They are practising creating scenarios in their minds and becoming active creators in life rather than training to be passive recipients. An environment where they can engage their right brains and where the parents do the same will facilitate this.

It's so important for children to have time outdoors in nature. Even later when they experiment with the artificial world they will have that basis of sanity in their minds.

Women

I want to share here something about women's hormonal situation in particular. It's about alleviating oestrogen dominance. Oestrogen dominance is the phenomenon of there being too much oestrogen compared to progesterone. It's a result of the anomalous situation we are in is along with the other hormone imbalances such as lack of melatonin. Oestrogen dominance is an increasing problem even for young women and as women go through the years, this imbalance, or 'oestrogen dominance', gets more extreme eventually producing the 'peri-menopausal' and 'menopausal' symptoms. To further compound things, in modern times we have the arrival of oestrogen mimicers, xenoestrogens, in chemicals in our environment, including plastics.

The unpleasant symptoms of oestrogen dominance/progesterone deficiency can include depression, anxiety, premenstrual syndrome and excessive bleeding, inability to maintain pregnancies, interference with thyroid function, menopausal symptoms and increased risk of reproductive cancers. You can research more symptoms online.

Fortunately there are some simple things we can do to alleviate these symptoms, by addressing the cause. Firstly use a natural progesterone cream. I recommend the one I use and know to be effective, Wellsprings Serenity cream. By rubbing a tiny amount onto varying fatty areas of the body for half the days of the cycle, progesterone levels are gradually restored.

Consuming maca in addition to using the cream can really make the difference. Maca is an adaptogen and tends to bring the body back into balance. Heavy periods have become normal for so many women but they can become lighter with the use of maca and/or natural progesterone cream. At first the effect of the maca can be to make things seem a little worse. Then in the next month it tends to stabilise and the month after that it can be much better. Persevere, you can get a detox and be a little wiped out initially with maca - just keep going.

In addition to all this it makes sense for us all to supplement melatonin levels, especially as we get older and the levels fall. It is anti-ageing and massively anti-oxidant and will help bring hormone levels into balance.

Leslie Kenton writes this about the effects of xenoestrogens "watch out for xenoestrogens. Oestrogen dominance in women and the drop in sperm count in men have come about for several reasons, the major one being the widespread use of oestrogen based oral contraceptives and the exponential spread of chemicals in our environment. Called xenoestrogens - oestrogen mimics - they are taken up by the oestrogen receptor sites in our bodies to throw spanners in the works."

Longevity

We are developing neurally until at least our fifties, almost certainly beyond, and definitely have the potential to be gaining maturity and wisdom. To be degenerating from our twenties clearly doesn't make sense. It's an anomaly. It's not in our DNA to age as fast as we do. There are several mechanisms involved. Of course there is wear and tear; we are not being as efficiently repaired as it would be if we were optimally functioning. There is also hormonal degradation which I have given a lot of attention to. The other major known factor is telomere loss.

The whole anomalous biochemical and neural situation is obviously the main problem. Then the drop in melatonin levels and surge of sex hormones without abundant plant biochemistry to modulate it at puberty compounds the situation. Another glitch concerns the telomeres. As I explained in chapter 4, after the embryo stage we are lacking the enzyme telomerase which is involved in the replacement of telomeres, the ends of the strands of DNA which protect it. When cells divide, telomeres are lost and without telomerase they don't regrow. Eventually the telomeres grow so short that the cells concerned die through senescence and cannot continue to divide and function. Obviously this causes degeneration.

The Hayflick limit is the number of times a normal human cell population will divide until cell division stops. Obviously it is limited by the lack of telomerase. It determines the maximum human life expectancy, given an ideal situation, for example long lived cultures on the planet who live in pristine surroundings. These people can live to up to 130 years of age. With telomeres replenishing the possible life span would increase.

Many mythologies tell us of a prolonged youthful, almost childlike state, we could call it extended juvenility or youth, and massively long lifetimes compared with what we experience now. Scientific research is beginning to shed more light on this. I think we innately know this and this is why we are so keen to maintain our youth.

What are the answers? Obviously getting back into our ideal nutrition and supplementing to readjust the hormonal balance are the basis. Working on maintaining ideal hormonal levels as we grow older is also part of the picture. We want the sex hormone levels to remain at a healthily high level yet balanced with plant and pineal biochemistry. Then there is the reactivating of telomerase. Stem cell therapy and other treatments are beginning to emerge as ways to regenerating damaged parts. Long term of course, if the DNA is read according to its original blueprint, we can live our optimal lifespan, and, with the exalted state we would be in we would have a wholehearted desire to do so.

Death

In our disconnected state it's possible to have little sense of life beyond our lives and this makes death seem more frightening and more like a final ending. Indigenous cultures have a connection to the ancestors and life beyond death so it is perceived differently. This is where plant medicines have been so helpful to comfort people in the last part of their lives and assist the passage, also to help those still here connect with the ancestors. Psylocibin has been great help to people with terminal illnesses. The problem as usual is our state of consciousness, it's something that troubles us at every stage of life. Living in nature according to our true natures, death is a more seamless process and an entry into the next phase, rather than a battle to stay alive as long as possible. What most of us seek is quality of life and even youthfulness to live a productive, active life as long as is possible and then a peaceful dignified transition with a sense of connection to what lies beyond. With enhanced state of consciousness communication with the ancestors and those close who have passed over is a natural state of affairs. Even now this experience is regularly reported. How enriched would our lives would be and how much healthier would our culture be if we were to experience more of this.

On the subject of death, we are at a time of closure at this point of the human story because so much of what is happening is unsustainable and so much is being destroyed. For example, over half the animal population of the world has been lost since 1970 and looking at the epidemics in degenerative disease and also the escalation of war one wonders about the future for humans populations. The ability to transition through death is very relevant. There is something very beautiful about tying up loose ends knowing that new seeds have been sown. Birth and death are opposites, not life and death. However long we can live, it does seem that we are mortals and being able to have a real and positive sense of life beyond our lives is essential to living life to the full. After this sobering thought we now continue to live life to the full with some practical advice about delicious food preparation.

10. Recreating the Psychoactive Forest ~ in your Kitchen

This chapter is about replicating as far as possible the biochemistry that was ours in our original biological habitat the tropical forests. Using foods that are natural and beneficial to us to eat, not surprisingly create the most delicious recipes that not only give us health but also an incredible sense of wellbeing.

The Art of Tasty Food Preparation

In our pristine natural state with our senses fully alert, and our food fresh from the trees and ground we would experience orgasmic taste sensations. This was our original cuisine, the rightness of the food for us and our heightened senses. Cultural cuisines have developed to add this spice back into our lives. There are five tastes to be aware of to stimulate every part of your tongue and round out the flavours to turn your preparation from food into a delicious recipe. I'll come back to these shortly. You'll see that in the recipes I share with you generally at least four out of these five tastes are deliberately enhanced with particular ingredients.

Raw recipes are great as a starting point when entering into the new territory of raw food preparation. When you get the hang of the different methods and how raw ingredients can be used you will almost certainly be inspired to create your own concoctions. Favourite cookbooks too become a treasure trove of ideas when you get into the flow of it. Cooked dishes are easy to replicate when you get used to translating cooked ingredients into raw. Just think about the textures and flavours that really hit the spot with that favourite dish. Usually it's very simple: cooked chickpeas become sprouted chickpeas, blanched almonds become soaked almonds. Substitute a very sweet fruit such as dates for sugar and avocado for eggs and cream. Sometimes its a simple case of a simple switch to the raw ingredient rather than a processed version. The recipes in this book will show you many other substitutions – pastry made from almond and date; sauces made with raw fruit plus dried fruit to thicken; burgers, breads and crackers set with ground seeds. I learned these methods from a variety of sources – the recipes here are combinations of my own inspiration and also inspiration from others – all designed to help make your experience of eating the foods of consciousness as enjoyable as possible. Many of the recipes were inspired by childhood favourite cooked dishes and I thought about how to replicate the texture and flavour. You can do the same. Using ingredients and methods I describe here you can translate your own favourite cooked meals.

As described earlier in this book nutrient rich neuroactive raw food nourishes the creative, intuitive part of us which is probably why when people start eating such brain activating food they seem to come up with so many amazing dishes. The recipes in this book are ones created and enjoyed by me and my family and friends over the years. I have my own favourite ingredients – ones that I feel are nourishing in some special way whilst maintaining that light raw feeling – these ingredients pop up again and again in my recipes – cherries, strawberries, almonds and figs spring to mind. The recipes I create these days tend to centre around ingredients I know to have exceptionally beneficial qualities.

As our intuition becomes clearer by eating a natural diet, biochemical supplementation and conducive living habits we find our hands know the amounts of any ingredient to add to the blender - superfoods and seasonings are sprinkled in. It's good to treat food preparation as a meditative practice, undistracted and focused on making food that is delicious and right for the people who are going to eat it, giving the people we are making food for the nutrients they need at that moment.

One of the wonderful things about raw recipe design is that you haven't got the unknown factor of the cooking process to take into account – you can just keep adding the ingredients until it tastes right. This has liberated the inner chef in many people. I have found this especially helpful with spices - you can easily adjust the amounts to taste without wondering what it will taste like when it's cooked. The amounts given in the recipes here are for guidance. The only major factor to be aware of is that when you add thickeners such as psyllium or flax seeds they absorb flavour as well as moisture and this is particularly noticeable with dehydration. Sauces made with dried fruit such as sun-dried tomatoes, dried mango or cherries or nuts such as macadamias will set a while after you make them.

One of the joys of raw food preparation is the absence of clock watching. There are no oven times – just chop or blend or leave in the fridge until it's the right consistency for you. You can break off to do something else you need or want to do and there aren't the stress of things getting burnt !

Let your imagination carry you. A clean kitchen, filled with the life of growing plants and sprouting seeds, a botanical tea, incense, or your music of the moment all help get that right brain engaged and immerse us in an awareness of physical reality. Personally I don't like to talk while I am making food for that reason – I want peace so that I can put love into the food I am making. At the end of the day, it's that presence, that concentration on the matter in hand that produces the results and is the secret of making delicious food. One of the great things about eating this way is you don't have to spend a lot of time in food preparation if you don't want to. Raw food is the original fast food and you can if you wish, keep it to simple smoothies, drinks, fruit and salads and so forth.

Emotional transference

After a while eating this way, recipes that mimic cooked dishes often taste far nicer than the original cooked version. When I tried my favourite cooked tomato soup recipe again after a few months eating raw food I was shocked how little it tasted like my memory – the real thing was now my raw tomato soup recipe. Maybe this is because raw foods are so much more alive and real. Then also I wonder if many cooked dishes were devised to mimic the ancient tastes of whole live foods such as the exotic fruits we would have found in our original habitats. Food tastes very different according to the state of your body. When you change eating habits an an emotional transference takes place and you start to get comfort from the new food. Easing this emotional transition is one reason why so many raw dishes are created in the likeness of, and named after, cooked counterparts – to stimulate fond memories and keep connection with our roots. As time goes on and your tastes readjust you may find yourself preferring the taste of whole natural foods such as a simple fruit or vegetable. This happens naturally so enjoy raw cuisine and make it fun.

Tastes

There is an art to making a delicious dish that is more than a plate of food one that is a complete taste experience. Wild natural food has all the components of taste, but until our full sense of taste returns we cannot always appreciate it. Including the full taste spectrum of sweet, sour (acid), salt, fatty (oily) and pungent explicitly in a dish makes all the difference.

Sweet: can be fruit, maple syrup, honey, stevia, sweet potato or other vegetable, coconut juice for example
Sour: this is an acidic taste for example, lemon, lime, orange, cider vinegar or even something as mild as apple or tomato.
Salt: sea salt or another natural salt or even a salty vegetable such as celery, alternatively miso or tamari
Fatty: a fatty fruit such as avocado, olives or an oil, or cream
Pungent: can be a strong tasting herb or spice or something with a strong aroma such as cacao.

Balanced Meals

These are some of the factors that make a balanced meal, that our bodies want inside them and makes us feel good afterwards.

A good mix of flavours as above i.e. presence of sweetness, saltiness, fat, acid and a distinctive flavouring ingredient.

Alkalinity - a healthy body is alkaline overall and the body will take whatever minerals it needs to keep our blood alkaline so we survive. Our food is far more nutritious therefore if it predominates in alkalising ingredients. Most fruit and vegetables are near the neutral mark even if they are alkaline. Green and citrus fruits stand out as being particularly alkalising and counteract the acid-forming foods in our diets such as nuts, seeds and grains. Almonds are an exception in that they are an alkalising nut. Raw dairy products are generally alkalising but not as much as greens or citrus. The presence of alkalising ingredients e.g. greens, celery, citrus fruit or other alkaline fruit transforms a meal.

A reasonably low glycemic index is helpful. It means that sugar is released into the blood stream at a manageable rate. You don't need to have measuring equipment! It can be achieved by using non-sweet and low-glycemic fruits or mixing protein and fatty foods with any high sugar fruits present to slow down the sugar release. Something I have noticed over the years is that when the brain is switched into a truly higher gear, in an exalted state of consciousness, presumably a state nearer to what our tropical forest dwelling ancestors would have experienced, fruit sugar is more easily used as a fuel and can be used up in larger quantities. Unfortunately in our current situation we as humans vary in our capacity to use fruit sugars as brain fuel. It is now believed that this could even be connected to dementia in some older people. In the situation of some degenerative diseases nutritional ketosis, i.e., reducing carbohydrate consumption to a small amount so that fat is the primary fuel used can have a therapeutic role.

If there are animal products i.e. raw dairy products involved they are generally in minimal quantities – the emphasis remains on the raw plant foods which are the pristine sources of nutrition.

The meal is all or nearly all fresh, raw ingredients. The more truly fresh the ingredients are the better we will feel. Freshness and life force are key. Living foods such a sprouts and kefir have a noticeable effect. Freshly picked greens and fruit have an impact way beyond store bought. Raw products in jars and packets are great savers when nothing else is available but cannot compare to freshly produced foods. For example seeds that have been soaked will have more life force than unsoaked seeds. If you then process them they are going to be in far better condition eaten straight after processing then a few hours or even days later. Frozen fruit especially berries though can be useful. Freezing does not damage food the way cooking does and sometimes you will even get fresher food this way.

The more wild or wild strain or heirloom variety ingredients, the better it feels.

High quality complete protein (a full range of essential amino acids) is part of the meal. It provides the materials for those all important neurotransmitters and satisfies our hunger.

The key to food combining is to think about how quickly a food take to digests and eat quick digesting foods such as fruit first. Melon should be eaten alone. Fruit should be eaten before other foods. Fruits and seeds naturally combine because seeds grow inside fruits.

Equipment

What equipment do we need? Here is the basic list:

Knife, chopping board and grater
A ceramic knife is ideal (but not essential) because it avoids refined metal coming into contact with the food.

A blender has a multi-prong arrangement and is good at breaking down liquid mixtures. It assists our digestive systems in breaking down food so we can absorb nutrients and save our energy. It also makes delicious combinations of food. High power ones such as Vitamix give smoother result and can break down unsoaked dried fruit, but a cheap one will do the job. This is the second piece of equipment to invest in after a good knife. If I could choose one piece of equipment I would choose a high power blender. They are expensive but go on year after year with intensive use, you don't have to soak dried fruit, they make fine creamy mixtures and make it possible to make dishes such as ice-cream. They blend green leaves finely in a way that other blenders cannot and make delicious creamy soups. A cheap blender (they can now be found very cheap indeed online) is fine for getting started.

A grinder is invaluable for breaking down nuts and seeds and making snacks and is inexpensive. A coffee grinder will do the job.

To break down more solid mixtures you need a food processor. A food processor has a twin blade. A high quality processor like a Magi-mix is ideal here for a fluffy smoothness but any processor will work. Powerful processor again means you don't have to pre-soak items such as sun-dried tomatoes and dried fruit, it gets through challenging stuff like grains and it will go on year after year but again, a cheap one is all you need to get started.

A dehydrator is basically a box with a fan at the back that blows warm air over food to warm and dry it. It contains a thermostat to make sure the food does not overheat. They are very useful for drying soaked seeds and nuts, making breads and replicating some cooked dishes. Its something to buy when you are ready. They can help immensely in the transition to eating more raw foods.

A juicer is useful obviously for juices, also for homogenising seeds, nuts and grains. I would not put it at the top of my list simply because I prefer to blend whole fruit and vegetables and it is possible to make juice if needed by putting this mixture through a muslin bag. It is something to buy when you feel inclined.

A vegetable peeler is useful for creating imitation spaghetti and pasta out of vegetables. Courgette served this way tastes very different to straight courgette – you may be surprised. Sweet potato works well too. There are spiralizers on the market that do this job in a fancy and fun way and will spiral slice in different ways for different vegetables. This is not essential, just fun and a great encouragement to eat vegetables in place of pasta made of grains.

Electronic Kitchen Scales are needed to follow exactly some of the recipes in the book and they can be purchased reasonably cheaply – Salter do some reasonably inexpensive models. If you don't have them you can judge many of the amounts by ingredients packet sizes and common sense.

A measuring jug is needed again for measuring ingredients and handling liquids.

A set of measuring spoons is helpful for measuring small amounts of ingredients.

Methods of Raw Food Preparation

Here's an explanation of the main preparation methods involved in raw cuisine.

Chopping, mashing, dicing and slicing you know.

Blending in the recipes means combining and breaking down of food with a blender until smooth.

Processing means breaking down and/or combining foods in a twin blade food processor.

Soaking is simply putting dry seeds, nuts or fruit in spring water to soften them and also break down phytates and growth inhibitors in seeds and nuts which would otherwise impair our assimilation of nutrients. This removes substances that aren't ideal for us and also brings them to life and makes them easier to digest. It's usually most convenient to soak things overnight but if you're in a hurry you can soak food for a couple of hours or so in warm water. Add fresh warm water from time to time to keep the temperature up and of course make sure it's not over body temperature. Soak water from fruit is lovely to use in recipes and to make nut and seed milks but soak water from seeds and nuts is best thrown away.

Grains such as kamut or spelt wheat need longer and warmer soaking than seeds and nuts. In summer room temperature is warm enough, but on cold days it may be necessary to warm the soak water and replace with fresh warm water at intervals.

Marinating is soaking raw ingredients in sauces and seasonings that will add flavour or break them down into a form that is more enjoyable to eat. This is a way of giving raw foods a similar texture to cooked. A combination of something acid, e.g. lemon juice, something salty, e.g. sea salt and something oily, e.g. olive oil will do the trick.

Thickening and setting can be achieved with seeds such as flax and psyllium, nuts such as macadamias, and coconut and dried fruit such as figs, apricots, sun-dried tomatoes, dried mangoes and dried montmorency cherries.

Grinding is used in many recipes and is done with foods such as dried nuts, seeds, cacao and bee pollen.

Grating is useful to make root vegetables such as raw carrots and sweet potato appealing. It makes foods taste surprisingly different to whole or sliced.

Dehydrating in a dehydrator is a method that has many uses. It can be used to dry out fruits such as tomatoes, to melt fats such as cacao or coconut butter and to warm food. It can be used to intensify the flavour of nuts by soaking the nuts, for example walnuts or pecans then dehydrating them. In pecans, in particular, it gives them that intensity of flavour usually brought out by cooking. It also means that even if we need dried nuts in a recipe we can soak them first to break down the growth inhibitors.

In the early days of making raw dishes this way we used to set the temperature to body temperature (about 100 degrees Fahrenheit) so as to avoid the risk of overheating the food (dehydrators are usually gauged in Fahrenheit which is still used in the USA). Recipes would often take many hours to dry out and moulds would sometimes develop on them soon after making because the temperature and moist atmosphere were ideal for their development. It was then realised that better results were achieved by setting the dehydrator temperature higher. The food does not reach the full temperature of the dehydrator, in the same way as food in an over does not reach the same temperature as the oven. The dehydrating and/or warming takes place quicker and mould growth is inhibited. Around 115 degrees Fahrenheit seems to work best but with very wet foods you can begin higher. The evaporation of the moisture keeps the temperature of the food down and as it dries out you can lower the dehydrator temperature.

Warming can be done in a dehydrator which will regulate the temperature. Soups can be warmed on a very low heat in a thick saucepan stirring continuously. You can use your finger to gauge the temperature and make sure it doesn't go above body temperature. If you keep dishes at or below body temperature or 40 °Celsius they remain raw or living foods.

Melting is usually in connection with chocolate making where the cacao butter needs melting. Break the cacao butter into as small pieces as you can or grate it. Put it in a container in a dehydrator until it has melted or put it in a small bowl in a larger container of fairly hot water.

In some of the recipes ingredients such as fruit and nuts are given in volumes, for example 250ml. This seems a bit unusual at first but is a very easy way of recording amounts. To measure ingredients this way just pile them in a measuring jug until they reach the level stated. Of course they don't fill out the jug the way liquids do but this is taken into account in the recipe. We are used to volume measuring using measuring spoons. Abbreviations used in the recipes in this book are:
tsp = teaspoon
Tbsp = tablespoon

Many blended recipes can be successfully frozen. Freezing does damage the structure of the food but not as much as cooking does. Delicious creamy ice creams can be made using bananas which have been peeled, broke into pieces and frozen overnight, then blended with other fruits and ingredients.

The Art of Foraging

Wild foods have strength and independence, flourishing effortlessly without effort by humans. They are varieties that can defend themselves against disease and pests, that are integrated into the surrounding ecology. Wild foods are perhaps they only true natural foods, unhybridised and unaltered. All wild foods are psychoactive – they energise the brain. They seem to possess an electricity and vibrancy beyond cultivated food. Wild foods have an energy of of their own, often growing on soil that has never been cultivated they are nutritionally superior especially in terms of minerals.

Raw is only the first part of the story, fresh is another. As our bodies and sensibilities refine themselves on a raw diet we notice how deteriorated much of the food available to us is, and the innate longing to eat food straight from the ground and trees returns. The life in this food gives us a completely different experience than food that has been stored for any length of time.

 Wild foods in temperate climates are very often not our original food species. Eating a good variety lessens the impact of any substances in them that are slightly toxic to us. Wild greens contain strong compounds and we are not meant to eat too much of one plant. As we move into warmer climates the experience is something else and we can enjoy, wild and fresh, the foods that are natural to us to eat. In Britain the berries are probably the most enjoyable wild edibles especially of course the blackberries and wild strawberries. One tiny wild strawberry seems to contain the entire experience of one large cultivated strawberry.

Edible varieties of greens include wild garlic leaves, violet leaves, pennywort, yellow archangel, cleavers, hawthorn leaves, bramble buds, gorse flowers, dandelion leaves, garlic mustard, crow garlic, rose garlic, nettles and dead nettle. Flowers include wild garlic, borage flowers, rose petals, evening primrose, dandelion and violet flowers. Let yourself be drawn to an appealing leaf or flower; tuning into the plants and countryside is as beneficial part of this experience as the eating of it. And take just a little from each area and walk to different places. A good rule of thumb until you get into the feel of it is to take up to 10% of a plant, or 10% of the leaves , fruits or flowers in an area. In time you may notice that you know exactly what to pick.

When you set out, be cautious with plants you do not know - some plants are dangerously poisonous e.g hemlock (easily confused with cow parsley), lords and ladies, some mushroom species. Never eat anything you are not sure about and preferably get a wild food expert in your area to show you around and identify both edible and poisonous plants.

The Art of Gardening

The relationship between the plants that we eat and ourselves is one of the most paramount ones in our lives. Even if we can only grow a little of our own food, even some sprouts or parsley on the window sill, a seed tray of sunflower sprouts in compost, one fruit tree or a pot of festuca grass or basil it will enhance the quality of our lives, it will connect us to the consciousness of life and give us a chance to feel more of that innate symbiotic connection with plants. It's been postulated that when we grow food for ourselves the plants will provide more of the nutrients we need, because of this innate connection.

Russia is interesting. With only 110 days growing season, 70% of the Russian population grow their own food in gardens (dacha) and 54% of all food in Russia is grown in backyard gardens using 7% of the agricultural land. What is more, the dachas are mainly on marginal lands with poor quality soil. There is an explanation for the greater productivity of the dachniks or dacha owners - the plants are better attended to because the growers are nearer to them. They only have from mid-May to mid-September to do all the growing and preserving of food. How much more could those of us living in lighter, warmer climates do!

In order to gain the most benefit from the gardening experience then the first priority is to reconnect to nature and the environment. The second is to make our plot beautiful. The third is to provide for our needs and this will be follow as a by-product of the first two. When we are connected to the environment and in a state of mind to see beauty we are actually functioning better and we will go about the food growing process in a more apt and intelligent way.

Eating local foods is of course important, yet to eat the requirements of our biological species also means for most of us including imported foods. It's a compromise. Of course growing our own food allows us the experience of eating freshly gathered food and incorporating heirloom, the more natural varieties and wild varieties into our gardening gives us a more complete experience. We may also find that with skill we can grow some of the non-native varieties of plants that are part of our original biological diet, for example, figs. We survive and flourish outside our biological habitats and, with our care, sometimes they can too.

Travel

A semi nomadic life is natural to humans that's why so many of us love traveling. The coming of agriculture tended to make us more settled but now, with modern communications and digital storage devices it's easy to travel and take our work and life with us. Wisdom is in the Earth and when we travel to different places we learn and develop in ways that would not be possible otherwise.

Traveling with biological nutrition is easy now too. It's always been possible to buy fruits and vegetables but now even cafes, service stations and food stands etc are far more likely to offer a salad, selection of fruit or other suitable meal. Superfoods, herbs and supplements can be easily packed into luggage. A small blender such as a nutribullet is another helpful thing to carry, also a small earthing pad or sheet. Dried foods that can be very useful are probiotic dried green powders, noni powder, vanilla powder, maca, lucuma, shilajit, MSM, sea salt, dried seaweed, and seeds. Kefir in bottles is surprisingly easy to travel with. It's possible to get raw cheeses in many places too. It's just a matter of thinking though how you will cover nutritional needs when traveling. Of course take any usual supplements and consider adding in a good essential fatty acid formula and coconut oil.

A good first aid kit includes (depending on where you are traveling if course) colloidal silver, tea tree oil, sangre de draco, citronella (to keep mosquitos away), lavender essential oil and coconut oil.

Bonus for those in temperate latitudes ~ Don't you feel cold in winter?

When I first got into raw food I was astonished that I could tread out into the white snow in bare feet and without feeling uncomfortable. I started to feel in winter the way I felt in summer. I concluded that much of the bad feeling of winter was more to do with winter eating and living habits than the actual weather.

As well as stodgy food, potential disconnection from nature and lack of exercise by staying indoors there are of course two major hazards associated with winter – lack of light and lack of warmth. These are real biological concerns for our species. We could be said to be designed for a life in the tropics or sub-tropics where the amount of light, warmth and tropical fruit is ideal for us. However, as a supremely adaptable species we are capable of flourishing in a wide variety of circumstances if we put our minds to it.

Raw food does not need to be cold! There is no reason at all not to have warm foods and liquids, if they are not heated above about 40 degrees Celsius their goodness and structure still remains intact. In Mediterranean countries food is traditionally often eaten this way anyway.. In our natural environment our food would all be slightly warm anyway so it would seem to be an ideal way to consume it. Warm superfood elixirs and vegetable soups can be made by using herbal teas as a base or even heating very carefully over a low heat. The key point is to keep the food at or below 'biological temperature' which is around 40 degrees celsius or the temperature of your body. Above that temperature the actual structure of some of the nutrients can begin to change. Dehydrators are another way of warming food if you like more solid foods. Spices such as cayenne and ginger boost the circulation and help keep us warm.

Coconut butter/oil and creamed coconut are great ingredients because they support the thyroid and therefore boost metabolism, helping us produce more energy and heat. Iodine is important for the function of the thyroid too and most of us lack it. This is largely because of depletion of mineral levels in the soil, the minerals have been effectively swept out to sea, sea vegetables and particularly kelp are some of the best sources.

We need to be cautious about habitually eating large amounts of cruciferous vegetables raw because they contain goitrogens, compounds which interfere in the uptake of iodine by the thyroid. However small amounts of goitrogens may have a beneficial health effect if balanced by ample amounts of iodine in the diet. Examples of cruciferous vegetables include kale, spinach, broccoli and cabbage. In traditional diets they were often fermented which introduces helpful probiotics.

Animals who live in cold climates and fish who swim in cold waters have a high percentage of omega 3 fatty acids in their bodies, and in the case of animals, especially in their feet. Many people notice that when the weather gets colder they are drawn to foods that contain these oils.

Omega 3's are polyunsaturated fats which stay liquid at low temperatures and it would seem that they help our bodies function in these circumstances. Seed oils such as those of flax and hemp and also fish liver oils are examples. It seems like we need denser foods in general in winter to compensate for the lack of warmth and sunshine in the outside world. If you think about it the energy, nutrients and genetic life information are stored in the seeds of plants during the winter season, ready to sprout forth in the spring. Along similar lines, 'medicinal' mushrooms such as reishi, lion's mane, chaga, tremella and cordyceps feel particularly good in winter and help our immune system. The dried mycelium powders (mycelia are the underground or root-like portions of the mushrooms) are delicious in marinades, dehydrated breads and elixirs. Herbs which boost the immune system also include echinacea, ginseng, garlic, astragalus and cat's claw.

Emotional comfort is important too. There are plenty of raw food snacks we can make and now buy in winter that will help us get through. Green powders such as barley grass, chlorella and spirulina can make up for the reduced availability of salad and wild greens and also help us keep alkalised if we are eating more nuts and seeds than in summer.

Personally I am for keeping ourselves as physically warm enough as we want to be when we are indoors. Below 28 degrees Celsius our bodies go into a mild form of stress maintaining our body temperature. By keeping warm we are allowing our parasympathetic nervous system to operate which means that both our bodies and brains function better. It may be more practical to keep just one part of our dwelling super warm

Light is a nutrient too. It seems that we assimilate food quite differently when we are in sunshine. Most people notice that they eat differently in sunny hot places than in cold places. There are many clues about this by looking at the traditional diets of people around the world, for example in the work of Dr Weston Price which I have mentioned. Basically, the further away you go from the equator, the higher percentage of animal foods including dairy products were traditionally included in the diet. It is as if when we moved away from our biological habitat we had to use the resources of species who could assimilate nutrients from plants that grew there, function successfully in the lower levels of sunlight, and could live unclothed outdoors to make use of the light there is. One of the factors involved is so-called fat soluble vitamins. They are principally vitamins A, D and K, which although found in plants, are only in the form we can use them in animal products such as dairy. These vitamins are essential for the body to actually make use of minerals such as calcium. Of course we can get vitamin D from sunshine but the fact is that between about September and March in the British Isles, the sun is too low to shine UVB light on our skins to make vitamin D. So – either we need to eat vitamin D rich foods or use a supplement. Sun-showers (a kind of stand up cubicle version of a sun-bed which emits carefully regulated doses of UVB) are also helpful if there is one in your area. Of course many people find that full-spectrum lighting really helps them maintain a good mood throughout the darker months.

Charge up with the Earth's electricity not the artificial electrical mains! It is tempting in winter to hole up indoors but actually if you can get out for a brisk walk in nature, even the local park, we are going to feel a whole lot better. Of course regular exercise improves our metabolism and makes us feel significantly warmer. It also helps us generate the feel-good brain chemical serotonin out of the amino acid tryptophan, get the lymphatic system moving and boost endorphin levels. We need connection with nature for mental well-being and, hesitant though I am to mention it, barefoot connection with the earth is as beneficial to us in winter as it is in summer.

On this note, I have noticed a strong if subtle difference to my experience in winter through wearing natural fabrics such as hemp, linen, organic cotton, bamboo and wool. They seem to help us keep a connection with the natural life force, the connection we take for granted in summer when we automatically tend to expose bare skin to the elements. Living structure has a pattern based on a ratio named the golden ratio which allows energetic information to flow freely through their material.

11. Succeeding ~ Bringing the Life Force Back into your Life

Here are some concluding thoughts on implementing the material in this book and the journey forward.

Success can be measured in many ways. One classic definition is the progressive realisation of a worthy goal. I like this way of looking at things because it implies that being on track is our measure of success, we are not required to reach some arbitrary point of perfection. Success in the terms of Food for Consciousness is a feeling. It's a feeling of fulfilment, of living your true life story, of being connected to source. It acknowledges that there are many challenges in the world today so we are not required to be in some perpetually blissed out state but to enthusiastically register the full range of emotions. Enthusiasm is the key word, it's what lifts us out of dull states into a passion for living. Should success spill over into a degree of financial and worldly success then it is firmly rooted in a sensation that we are being true to our destiny, that we are seen by forces bigger than us, that we aligned with benign supernatural forces, that we are engaged with the life force itself. Our lives become bigger than us.

This is a way of life that makes sense for anyone who wants a future on the planet.

Emotional

When we stop eating numbing foods and engaging in numbing life habits we feel a lot more. Developing an ability to deal with emerging inner conflicts and old issues will be part of the journey.

Social

Our success depends on also being able to integrate it into our existing lives but also into family life and social situations. This is increasingly less of a problem as so many people are seeing the benefits of healthy lifestyle. To be honest the time has come for this change. With delicious recipes to share it never really has to be a problem, especially if you are a shiny example of the benefits without foisting it on anyone else. People are sensitive to possible judgement of their own lifestyles.

Nutritional

Getting in enough nutrients is crucial. If we don't we are likely to reach out for foods that will set us off kilter. It's easy to underestimate the amount of nutrition we genuinely need as malnourishment has become normalised amongst humans. As already mentioned, Katherine Milton's studies on primates indicate the level of nutrition we are actually aiming for in order to feel right in ourselves... It is natural for us to crave fats and sugars and if we don't get the natural form for our species from fruit and vegetables, seeds and nuts and raw animal fats and so forth or equivalents we will reach out for the food we encounter in the modern world, which is often junk food.

Five Good Habits

1. Set boundaries around what you feel comfortable with, then you see the beauty in life.
2. Don't wait until you are perfect to do something.
3. Take moments to stop and reflect.
4. Celebrate what others have and aspire and work to have what you would like in your life.
Develop your sense of identity through contact with nature.

This list comes from an interview with New York Times best selling author Glennon Doyle Melton where she discusses her discoveries about the habits shared by successful women.

Identity

A lot depends on choosing our sense of identity. Then setting ourselves targets that we can achieve. Getting grounded physically, and into your destiny, moving to your highest desires, and living your dream as part of the bigger dream; this is real success. The world lights up, life becomes magic and you move in the mystery of life.

We have the knowledge now to turn things around for humanity. A very happy story indeed for those who choose it. Setting our sights on what is possible for us we are already on the way there.

12. Recipes

Here are over 130 tried and trusted recipes. Nearly all of them are quick and simple ones, all of them are easy to make at home. Some of them, in particular a few of the dessert recipes, are a bit more elaborate and probably for occasional use. After a while most people find that their bodies acclimatise to eating mostly fresh salads, fruit, simpler more liquid blends and possibly some simple cooked foods for every day use and the gourmet dishes remain a valuable way of celebrating or sharing healthy food with family and friends. The recipes I have continued to use regularly day in day out are notably the Chocolate Pudding, smoothie and drink recipes. Elaborate salads have continued also to be a way of life. Most of the ingredients can be bought in greengrocers, supermarkets or health foods stores, or online.

Smoothies, Reset and Rejuvenation Recipes

These are great simple recipes to get started with. These liquid blended recipes are ideal to include as part of a cleansing and super-nourishing reset protocol. These are recipes I use myself in cleansing programs both for myself and with clients.

Cherry Lemonade

250g sour cherries (can be frozen ones)
1 litre coconut water
dash sea salt
3 lemons with outer peel removed or 1 lime and 1 orange
3 tablespoons olive oil or 6 tablespoons soaked chia seeds/1 tablespoon coconut oil

Blend together until smooth.

Tropical Shake

250g mixed pieces of mango, pineapple and papaya
1 litre coconut water
juice of 2 limes
½ tsp vanilla
dash salt

Blend ingredients together.

Berry Smoothie

250g mixed berries (can be frozen)
2 bananas
1 teaspoon dried noni powder
½ teaspoon vanilla powder
½ litre coconut water/seed milk

Blend all ingredients together

Seaweed Soup

25g dried seaweed, for example wakame
1 clove garlic
1 tablespoon coconut oil
juice of 1 lemon
1 teaspoon curry powder
3 cups water/warm chaga tea or other herbal tea
1 tsp umeboshi paste

dash sea salt

Blend the ingredients together well and serve warm.

Sweet Potato Soup

3 medium sweet potatoes chopped or grated
250ml coconut milk from blending coconut juice and flesh of young coconut
½ red onion chopped
red pepper chopped
dash salt
1 lemon juiced
ginger 1 cm cube, grated
garlic 1 clove, crushed
curry powder to taste

Blend all the ingredients together.

Warm and Raw Miso Soup

3 Tbsps raw miso
juice of 2 lemons
garlic 1 clove, crushed
1 cm cube ginger root, grated
3 cups spring water, warmed

Blend ingredients together until smooth.

Gazpacho

3 medium tomatoes
½ cucumber
1/2 small onion
1/2 red pepper
1 garlic clove
1 avocado
1/4 lemon/lime juice
2 cup fresh water
1/2 chill
dash salt
herbs such as parsley coriander or basil to taste

Chop all ingredients and blend

Chocolate Elixir

For the tea:
2 Tbsps Pau d'Arco
2 Tbsps cat's claw
3 cups boiling water
let steep for 10 mins

Ingredients to add to tea base:
¼ tsp shilajit
½ tsp vanilla powder
2 tbs maca powder
honey to taste
40g creamed coconut/2 tablespoons coconut oil
pinch cayenne
pinch cinnamon

pinch nutmeg
pinch cardamom
1 Tbsps cacao powder

Pour tea base into blender.
Add remaining ingredients.
Blend until smooth and creamy.

Chocolate Pudding

This is a delicious recipe which provides comprehensive nutrition. People report it will keep them feeling energised all day. It is in the Breakfasts section.

Seed Milks

Hemp Milk

150g hemp seeds soaked overnight in water
200 – 300ml liquid – this can be all water or freshly squeezed orange juice, dried fruit soak water or a mixture of these. 1 orange gives about 50ml juice.

Drain the hemp seeds and blend with the liquid until the hemp seeds are broken down and the liquid looks milky.

Strain and squeeze through muslin or similar cloth to make hemp milk. A muslin bag is easiest.

Hemp milk should be consumed fresh and kept in the fridge for no longer than a day. The milk is exceptionally nutritious.

This milk can be added to sweet or savoury dishes or drank fresh as it is.

Other Seed and Nut Milks

You can make other nut & seed milks in the same way hemp milk above. Almond, hazelnut, sunflower, and sesame work well. Soak the seeds or nuts overnight as with the hemp seeds. In the case of almonds it's a good idea to remove the skins before making the milk because they contain a lot of tannin but it is time consuming and not crucial – much of tannin is taken out by the soaking anyway.

Other Drinks

Elderflower Cordial

1 ½ pints/800ml spring or filtered water
10 dried figs
Juice of ½ lime/lemon
4 or more sprigs of elderflowers

Soak figs and flowers in water with the lime juice overnight.
It ferments slightly and is very slightly fizzy

Elders flower in late spring or early summer.

Brain Wake Up Tea

For each person:

1 tsp rhodiola (rosea or kirilowii)
1 Tbsp ginkgo leaves
1 t tsp rooibosch (redbush) tea or 1 rooibosch tea bag
1 tsp tulsi tea

Simmer in water for five minutes.
Serve black or with raw milk.

Rhodiola creates mental alertness without the come down of caffeine. Boosts serotonin levels. Can keep you awake at night.
Ginkgo improves memory.
Tulsi relieves stress.
Rooibosch is rich in antioxidants and flavonoids. It is soothing yet also energising and also thirst quenching.

Breakfasts

Berry Smoothie/Jelly

1 banana
½ litre coconut juice
juice of 1 orange
1 tsp noni powder
½ tsp vanilla powder
¼ tsp schizandra powder
 300g frozen berries
1 Tbsp chia seeds soaked in spring water

Blend all the ingredients together until smooth.
If you leave in the fridge for a few hours it turns into jelly.

Chocolate Pudding

This delicious recipe was originally devised by Tony Wright, author of Return to the Brain of Eden, as a comprehensive neural system nourishment. I have embellished it a little. This recipe serves 3 or 4 people. It freezes successfully to become a supernutritious ice cream. This staple recipe is one I have used as a regular part of the nutritional routine for over a decade.

Basic ingredients:
1 recipe Hemp Milk made with 150g hemp seeds soaked overnight in water
200 – 300ml liquid (water or freshly squeezed orange juice, dried fruit soak water, or a mixture of these.   1 orange gives about 50ml juice)
a little orange zest
3 dried figs, soaked overnight in water
3 dried apricots, soaked overnight in water
50g sunflower seeds, soaked overnight in water
50g pumpkin seeds, soaked overnight in water
50g sesame seeds, soaked overnight in water
3 bananas
few chunks fresh coconut or 1 Tbsp coconut oil
a few grains Himalayan or sea salt
½ tsp vanilla powder
2 tsps cacao or cocoa powder

Optional extras/substitutions:
maca
algarroba
purple corn powder
hemp leaf powder
he shou wu
goji berries
blueberries, strawberries,
lime juice and zest
prunes instead of apricots
walnuts, hazelnuts, macadamias or brazils instead of some of the seeds

To make:
To make hemp milk, drain the hemp seeds and blend with the liquid until the hemp seeds are broken down and the liquid looks milky. Strain and squeeze through muslin or similar cloth to make hemp milk. A muslin bag is easiest.
Drain the soaked ingredients.
Blend all the ingredients together until smooth.
By the way if you are using a very powerful blender it may not be necessary to pre-soak the dried fruit – you then get a thicker result.

You can mix a tablespoon of flax oil into each person's serving increase the omega 3/omega 6 fatty acid balance.
This recipes is particularly delicious topped with fruit such as cherries, raspberries, mango and/or a little kefir or live yoghurt or ground hazelnuts.

Best Ever Strawberry Granola

150g almonds, soaked
75g sunflower seeds, soaked
150g fresh coconut
1 tsp mesquite powder
1 tsp maca powder
1 tsp rosehip powder
½ tsp vanilla powder
¼ tsp ground cinnamon
3 dried figs
3 dried apricots
2 Tbsp cold pressed honey
300g strawberries, sliced
2 pears, diced

Process together all the ingredients except the last two until broken down and smooth
Mix in the chopped fresh fruit.
Crumble the mixture over dehydrator sheets
Dehydrate until desired consistency. This is likely to be several hours and can be left on overnight.

Golden Crunch Cereal
by Jasmine Barratt

9 Tbsps raw rolled oats
5 Tbsps raw shredded coconut
1 Tbsp yacon syrup
4 Tbsp honey
4 ½ Tbsps sesame seeds
1 Tbsp bilberries
1 Tbsp currants
optional addition: 2 Tbsps bee pollen

Process all these ingredients together but not long enough to totally break down ingredients.

Press mixture onto dehydrator sheets and dehydrate still it starts to dry. Break up the mixture into breakfast cereal sized clumps and dry further. Store in sealed tub or bag.

Banana and Tahini

Bananas
Raw tahini

A simple combination – just mash 1 or 2 bananas per person with spoonfuls of tahini to taste.
You can blend – it gives a slightly different flavour and texture. This has remained a favourite breakfast in a hurry or snack for our family throughout.

Bananas dipped into tahini is also a delicious and filling combination. Raspberries go well with this mix, also carob or chocolate powder can be mixed in/

Seasonings

Chilli Oil

Fresh or dried chilli peppers
Cold pressed virgin olive oil

Chop chilli peppers and place in olive oil in a jar.
Effective as a seasoning within a few days if using fresh chillies or a couple of weeks if using dried chillies. If using fresh chillies keep in the fridge.
Keeps for a few weeks. Very hot!

Hot Curry Powder

6 tablespoons coriander seeds
1 ½ teaspoons cumin seeds
3 tablespoons turmeric powder
2 teaspoons black peppercorns
1 teaspoon fenugreek seeds
10 dry chilli pods
20 curry leaves
½ teaspoon cardamom seeds

Grind until fine and store in jar in cool dry place.

Green Juices

Superdelicious Green Juice

This combination of ingredients covers the five tastes and turns superhealthy ingredients into a delicious recipe. Obviously you don't need to include all of them.
beetroot
lemon or lime juice
apple
onion
sea salt
hemp seeds (soaked)
wild greens such as thistle, nettles, chickweed, plantain
ginger
cucumber
celery

Nettle, Carrot and Celery Juice

Nettles make a great juice because they are extremely nutritious, in terms of minerals, serotonin and mucus abilities. They are abundant and free, and mood lifting. Use nettles in spring before they flower because the composition changes at this time. Pick just the very top of the nettle. It's worth picking a couple of large bags of them as a small amount of concentrated juice is produced.

Nettles juice well with celery and carrot – the other vegetables give volume and improve the taste. If you put a celery stick through the juicer after the nettles, it clears those remaining valuable nettles.

Celery, like nettles, is very alkalising.

Carrot adds sweetness and contains the monatomic elements iridium and rhodium, important for brain function. The carrot pulp left after making juice is a useful cake ingredient, adding moisture, lightness and volume.

Soups

Raw soups can be gently heated and still remain equally nutritious as long as you don't heat them over biological or body temperature (about 40 degrees Celsius). Warm them on low temperature, stirring in a saucepan.

Cream of Tomato Soup

500g tomatoes
60ml olive oil
30ml lemon juice
basil to taste
sea salt to taste

optional:
2 tablespoons kefir or yoghurt to taste

Blend all the ingredients together until creamy.. This soup is delicious cold but if you like you can to warm it in a pan on minimum heat, stirring continuously until body temperature.

Hot Tomato Soup

Add a few drops of chilli oil to above recipe (see Chilli Oil recipe)

Lime, Coconut and Watercress Soup

100g watercress
1 avocado
1 tomato
3 halves sun-dried tomatoes
Juice of ½ lime
A little galangal if available
 A handful of basil leaves
Juice of 1 fresh coconut
10 x 1cm square pieces of fresh coconut
1 ½ pints water
Salt to taste

Blend until smooth.
If desired, warm carefully to body temperature in a saucepan, stirring all the while.

Creamy Carrot and Coriander Soup

1 kg carrots
10g fresh coriander
¼ teaspoon ground coriander
dash nutmeg
2 Tbsps live yoghurt (sheep's yoghurt is particularly good in this recipe)

Juice carrots and set aside pulp (it can be used for cake making e.g. Black Forest Gateau)

Blend the juice, herbs, spices and yoghurt until well mixed
If you would like it warm then heat gently in a thick saucepan on minimum heat, stirring all the while until body temperature
Serves 3

Miso soup

3 Tablespoons raw miso
juice of 2 lemons
1 clove garlic
ginger 1 cm cube
1 pint warm spring water

Blend all the ingredients together, serves 2

Basic Green Raw Soup

2 big handfuls green leaves such as watercress, rocket or wild greens and a little parsley and/or basil
1 large tomato
1 sun-dried tomato
1 stick celery
2 carrots
1 avocado
1 tsp green superfood powder
500ml water

optional extras:
½ bell pepper
¼ tsp mushroom powders e.g reishi, shitake
¼ tsp green algae

Blend all these ingredients together until smooth
Suggested toppings:
grated carrot
grated hard raw cheese
sprouts such as red clover, alfalfa, fenugreek

Watercress and Garlic Soup

1 big handful watercress
1 or 2 cloves garlic
2 tomatoes
1 sun-dried tomato
1 avocado
2 teaspoons or 10 ml flax oil
1 tablespoon or 15 ml lemon juice
1 ½ pints water

Blend all ingredients until smooth. A high-speed blender gives particularly creamy soup.

Alkalising soup with vegetable juice and cucumber

16 -20 oz/450-550 ml juiced celery, beet, onion, garlic, ginger and lemon
1 avocado
half a red bell pepper
half a cucumber (English)
pinch salt
pinch cayenne

Blend all ingredients and warm gently if desired

Garnish with some tasty dehydrated crackers, cubed raw goats cheese and alfalfa sprouts

Rich and warming soup made with tea

1 sweet potato
1 courgette
1 leek
60g creamed coconut
40g seaweed – wakame or sea spaghetti recommended
yogi or other tea
salt and pepper to taste

soak seaweed in tea
blend everything
serve with garnish of sprouts or yoghurt

See other soups in the Reset and Rejuvenation section

Savouries and Salads

Blended Salad

a couple of big handful greens e.g. watercress, mixed wild greens or other greens
2 tomatoes
2 sun-dried tomatoes
1 avocado
Dash lemon juice
dash salt
½ a cucumber
2 carrots

enough water to blend into soft consistency
optional:
150g pumpkin seeds
2 tsp miso

Blend, Serves 2
Especially in spring when I like to eat mountains of wild greens I often choose to blend my salad as its so much quicker and easier way to get all that nutrition in, and feel fantastic quickly.

Daily Salad

Make layers as follows:
LOTS of salad greens (wild when possible, if not then as near wild as possible such as rocket), finely chopped
handful alfalfa or red clover and fenugreek sprouts if I have made them
2 grated carrots or grated sweet potato
a handful parsley and/or basil finely chopped
3 large tomatoes chopped up
½ yellow pepper, diced
1 cucumber grated or diced
1 avocado, chopped or a handful of black or Kalamata olives

sprinkling sea salt, lime juice, olive oil and black pepper
100g unpasteurised goats cheese, diced and sprinkled on top
serves two

Creamy Cheese & Tomato Pasta

Tomato sauce:
8 medium tomatoes
8 halves sun dried tomatoes (soaked)

3 medjool dates, pitted
juice of 1 lime
2 tablespoons olive oil
sea salt to taste

Optional:
1 clove garlic
¼ red onion / 1 shallot, diced
fresh oregano and basil to taste

Blend all ingredients in a blender until fairly smooth but still a little chunky.

Pasta:
4 large courgettes

Use either a specific noodle type pasta maker or a vegetable peeler to make strips of pasta by continually peeling the courgettes over a bowl or simply grate.

Cheese topping:

One of the Cheese Sauce recipes below and if desired, 100 g finely grated raw cheese

1. Place pasta portion onto serving dish.
2. Top pasta with a portion of the tomato sauce.
3. Drizzle a portion of the cheese sauce on top of this.
4. Sprinkle grated cheese if desired.

Serves 4.

Cheese Sauce

50 g sunflower seeds
50 g macadamia nuts
50g pine nuts
2 Tablespoons yeast flakes
Salt & pepper to taste
Water

Optional:
50 – 100 g raw cheese (preferably soft)

Blend all ingredients with water (the amount will dictate consistency) until completely smooth.

This can be used in raw pasta dishes, or poured over chopped/grated vegetables.

Quick Rich Cheese Sauce

120ml water
60g pine nuts
60g unpasteurised hard cheese grated (parmesan or hard goat's work well)
A pinch paprika powder

Blend all the ingredients until smooth.

Delicious served with raw 'Fried' Mushrooms in the next recipe.

Fried Mushrooms

250g chestnut or other mushrooms, sliced
½ teaspoon Himalayan salt or sea salt
2 tablespoons olive oil
sprinkling lemon juice

mix and dehydrate for 30 minutes
optional:
put slices of unpasteurised goats cheese in at the same time to have melted cheese with them

Mushroom Spaghetti

Some of the ingredients for this dish are obviously a little unusual – you can find out where to get them in the suppliers.

30g sea spaghetti, soaked for 30 minutes
¼ cucumber
2 large flat or 6 medium mushrooms
pinch salt, diced and sprinkled with salt
1 tomato, diced
Sprinkling mushroom mycelium powder (Lion's Mane and/or tremella recommended)
¼ tsp crystal manna (optional but highly recommended)
15 – 30g raw goat's cheese, cubed

Dice the mushrooms and sprinkle with salt
Grate the cucumber
Mix mushrooms and cucumber with spaghetti and tomatoes, and then sprinkle mushroom powder and crystal manna or other blue green algae.

Cut the cheese into cubes and stir in.

This is a very satisfying raw meal.

Some of the ingredients for this dish are obviously a little unusual – you can find out where to get them in the suppliers.

Coconut Potato

1 large sweet potato grated
handful shredded coconut
handful fresh coriander
salt to taste

Mix together
Serve with salad greens, grated cucumber, a curry sauce and a little live yogurt

Corn and Sweet Potato in Coconut Sauce

2 corn on the cobs
2 Tablespoons olive oil
½ teaspoon cumin
1 teaspoon ground coriander seeds
½ teaspoon fennel leaves
pepper to taste
sea-salt to taste
chilli powder, chillies, or chilli oil to taste
1 teaspoon grated ginger
1 teaspoon curry leaves
½ teaspoon turmeric powder
10 almonds, soaked, peeled and chopped

flesh of one young coconut
coconut water to taste
1 sweet potato, grated
handful of coriander leaves, chopped

Cut corn off the cob
Process coconut, oil and spices
Mix corn, sweet potato, almonds and coconut mixture together
Add coconut water and coriander leaves to taste

This is based on an Indian recipe, substituting corn for pulses which many people find hard to digest. The original recipe contained mustard seeds but they have been omitted because they should not be eaten raw.

Thai Fried Rice

1 cauliflower
3 tablespoons flax oil
½ teaspoon turmeric
½ teaspoon ground cumin
¼ teaspoon ground cardamom
1 avocado, chopped
2 cloves garlic, crushed or grated
5 spring onions, chopped
small handful fresh coriander, chopped

Process cauliflower to rice like consistency. Mix in oil and spices. Stir in other ingredients.

Serve with Thai Green Curry Sauce and Asparagus

Falafels

280 g (1 cup/ ½ pint) chick peas, soaked overnight and then allowed to sprout for 24 hours (makes about 4 cups/ 2 pints)
2 cloves garlic
About 4 tablespoons fresh parsley
1 tablespoon dried cumin
1 tablespoon dried coriander
2 tablespoons lemon juice
dash salt to taste
sprinkling freshly ground black pepper to taste
3 tablespoons olive oil
2 teaspoons chilli oil or chilli powder to taste

Process all the ingredients together
Shape into 40gram balls
Dehydrate for a few hours, turning once, until outsides are crispy.

Seed Burgers / Cheese Burgers

The combination of seeds in this filling recipe is an excellent source of protein as it covers all the essential amino acids. Adding a layer of unpasteurised cheese makes it extra satisfying.

main ingredients:

30g pumpkin seeds, soaked
30g sunflower seeds, soaked
30g sesame seeds, soaked
90g shelled hemp seeds
8 sun-dried tomato halves
1 stick celery
1 floret broccoli

handful fresh parsley
salt and pepper to taste
1 tsp Provençal herbs (i.e thyme, rosemary, oregano, marjoram)
dash fresh lemon juice
optional extra: sprinkling of mushroom powders
½ red bell pepper

to set the burgers:
30g flax seeds
for cheeseburgers:
50g unpasteurised cheese, e.g. Gruyère

Drain the seeds and process with the rest of the main ingredients in a food processor.
Grind the flax seeds, add to the food processor and process the whole mixture until well combined.
Shape into six burgers and dehydrate until set (about 2 - 3 hours), turning half way through.
If making cheese burgers add a slice of cheese onto the top of each burger and leave in the dehydrator until the cheese softens.
These burgers go well with gherkins or cucumber and a fresh mixed salad of greens, grated carrot, and tomato. Chilli Sauce complements this recipe, adding moistness and intensity of flavour.. Serves three

Nut Roast

120g almonds, soaked overnight and drained
120g pumpkin seeds, soaked overnight and drained
60g sesame seeds, soaked overnight and drained
70g hazelnuts, soaked overnight and drained
70g walnuts, soaked overnight and drained
handful parsley

handful coriander
2 Tbsp lemon juice
1 tsp tamari
3 Tbsp nori
2 sticks celery, diced
3 florets of broccoli
6 sun-dried tomatoes soaked with juice of 2 oranges
1 Tbsp coconut oil
3 Tbsp flax seeds soaked with 3 Tbsp water for about 15 minutes

Process the nuts then add all the other ingredients and process together. Shape into a slab or portions about 1.5cm thick and dehydrate at about 115 degrees Fahrenheit, turning once until sides are crispy.

Purple Coleslaw
Vegetables:

500g red cabbage
200g sweet potato

Mayonnaise:

90ml olive oil
90ml flax oil or hemp oil
120ml grapefruit juice
4 tablespoons or 60ml unpasteurised miso

Shred the cabbage and grate the sweet potato
To make the mayonnaise, blend the oils, juice and miso and mix into the vegetables.

This combination of ingredients gives a beautiful purple and gold effect. Instead of sweet potato you can use another root vegetable such as carrot, turnip and parsnip also work well. You can substitute lemon juice or even orange juice for the grapefruit. These exact weights work well but you don't have to weigh the ingredients exactly - you can just stick in, say, ½ large cabbage and a largish sweet potato in and it will work out fine.

Real Risotto

1 cauliflower
2 tablespoons flax oil
1 teaspoon dried turmeric
1 teaspoon cumin
¼ teaspoon cardamom
3 spring onions, chopped
1 red or orange pepper, chopped

Optional:

1 shallot, chopped
crushed garlic
handful soaked sultanas
a few drops chilli oil

Process cauliflower until consistency of rice or couscous (not too much or it will change the flavour). Mix in oil, spices and other ingredients.
Serve with Savoury Orange Sauce, Orange Curry Sauce or Green Thai Sauce.

This dish goes well with banana, coleslaw, sun-dried peppers or .'Fried' Mushrooms (see recipe)

It is called Real Risotto in appreciation of how real to our system raw food is and how much our bodies appreciate it.

Savoury Sauces, Pates, Dips and Dressings

Savoury Orange Sauce

juice of 4 oranges
2 tablespoons olive oil
4 tablespoons unpasteurised miso

Blend until smooth.

This is goes well with 'Real Risotto' or grated vegetables, such as carrots or sweet potatoes on a bed of salad.

Orange Curry Sauce

Base:
1 recipe Savoury Orange Sauce
Spices:
2 teaspoons 'Hot Curry Powder'
or:
½ teaspoon cumin seeds
1 teaspoon coriander seeds
¼ teaspoon cardamom
1 teaspoon grated ginger
1 clove garlic

Grind the spice seeds unless using a high powered blender in which case there is no need to grind them separately.

Blend ingredients into sauce.

Coconut Curry

10 chunks of coconut (around 1cm square) or 20g coconut flakes
4 large tomatoes or 6 medium tomatoes
4 whole sun-dried tomatoes
2 slices dried mango
1 tablespoon Hot Curry Powder
sea salt or Himalayan salt to taste

Optional:
2 tablespoons or more kefir or raw yoghurt either blended into the sauce or served separately.

Blend all the ingredients together, adding a little water if necessary.

Serve with fresh green salad.

Chilli Sauce

3 large or 6 medium tomatoes
3 large sun-dried tomatoes
2 dried chillies
20g flaked coconut or fresh coconut
½ red pepper
15g dried mango

Optional, for more creaminess:
180 ml kefir/yoghurt or 1 avocado

Serve with green salad and grated root vegetables such as carrots

Green Thai Sauce

Main Ingredients:

4 oranges, juiced
2 tablespoons olive oil
4 tablespoons miso
2 teaspoons green superfood or a handful of watercress or wild leaves such as ramsons (wild garlic)

Herbs and Spices:

2 cloves garlic (if not using garlic leaves)
½ teaspoon ground coriander
½ teaspoon ground cumin
1 teaspoon grated ginger
small amounts of all or some of the following (whatever's available):
chilli/chilli oil
dill
galangal
caraway seeds (take care, they add bitterness)
basil/sweet Thai basil
kra chai (Thai ginger)
lime leaves
lime peel
lemongrass
fresh turmeric
fenugreek

Blend the main ingredients together then add the herbs and spices, blending in one at a time in small amounts until it tastes right.

This is nice served over asparagus.

Guacamole

5 avocados
5 tomatoes
1 onion diced
handful coriander, chopped up
dash salt
2 limes juiced

Mash all the ingredients together

Spicy Salsa

6 tomatoes
a handful of basil
1 Tbsp olive oil
dash sea salt
vinegar (Mexican pineapple vinegar if you can get it)
3 spring onions chopped up
1 clove garlic
dash paprika
dash chilli
1 Tablespoon honey

Blend all the ingredients together until desired consistency.

Mango Salsa

1 mango peeled and diced

1 small red onion finely diced
1 red chilli deseeded and diced
juice of one lime
grated zest of ½ a lime
3 Tbsp of finely chopped coriander
1 tbsp of finely chopped mint
sea salt to taste
freshly ground pepper to taste
1 clove finely chopped garlic

Combine all ingredients in a bowl and leave to sit for at least 15 minutes.

Garlic Pate

30g sunflower seeds, soaked overnight
30g pumpkin seeds, soaked overnight
30g hazelnuts, soaked overnight
2 small cloves garlic
pinch salt
sprinkling lemon juice

Blend all ingredients together.

Olive and Almond Pate

500g black or Kalamata olives, pitted
500g almonds, soaked overnight
90ml olive oil
juice of ½ lemon
3 cloves garlic

Process ingredients together until smooth.

This is nice wrapped with chunks of tomato in lettuce leaves.

Pesto
by Jasmine Barratt

Green Pesto
25g pine nuts
20g hard goat's cheese/parmesan
6 handfuls fresh basil
2 cloves garlic
1 date
3 tablespoons olive oil
juice of 1 lime
salt and fresh ground pepper to taste

optional:
6 drops mirin (Japanese cooking wine)

Red Pesto
add 9 halves sun-dried tomatoes

Wild Spring Pesto

A handful of wild garlic (ramson) leaves or watercress
A handful of basil
90ml freshly squeezed apple juice or orange juice
90ml olive oil
60g pumpkin seeds, soaked
salt and pepper to taste

Blend until smooth

This is very tasty served with courgette grated or spiral sliced.

Tomato Guacamole

3 avocados
2 large tomatoes
¼ red onion
1 tablespoon flax oil
5 sun-dried tomatoes, soaked
optional: a few drops chilli oil

Process ingredients together until smooth

Hummus

280g chick peas, soaked overnight and sprouted for 24 hours (makes about 2 pints)
4 cloves garlic
4 tablespoons raw white tahini or ground sesame seeds
1 teaspoon salt or 2 teaspoons tamari
5oz or 150ml lemon juice
30g parsley, chopped
30ml olive oil
30ml flax oil

optional extras:

6 sun-dried tomato halves
basil
wild garlic leaves (ramsons) to replace garlic not as strong

a few drops chilli oil
for a spicy hummus add sprinklings of paprika, cumin, turmeric and/or black pepper to taste.
Process, adding water if necessary, until smooth

Pumpkin Seed 'Cheese'

2 cups pumpkin seeds, soaked
2 cloves garlic
1 tsp grated ginger
1 tsp chilli oil
60 ml olive oil
30ml lemon juice
a few leaves wild garlic or 1 garlic clove
process all the ingredients together until smooth

Simple Salad Dressing

90ml olive oil
60ml lemon juice
salt and pepper to taste

Seasonings

Chilli Oil

Fresh or dried chilli peppers
Cold pressed virgin olive oil

Chop chilli peppers and place in olive oil in a jar.

Effective as a seasoning within a few days if using fresh chillies or a couple of weeks if using dried chillies. If using fresh chillies keep in the fridge.
Keeps for a few weeks. Very hot!

Hot Curry Powder

6 tablespoons coriander seeds
1 ½ teaspoons cumin seeds
3 tablespoons turmeric powder
2 teaspoons black peppercorns
1 teaspoon fenugreek seeds
10 dry chilli pods
20 curry leaves
½ teaspoon cardamom seeds

Grind until smooth and store in jar in cool dry place.

Breads, Crackers and Pizza

I feel compelled by authenticity to say here that the reason I include these recipes is that they are an improvement health wise on classic bread, cracker and pizza recipes. They are not the ultimate destination. I am a firm believer in improving things in sustainable steps. Transitioning to a high raw diet has a momentum of its own. You can feel carried by the increasing sense of vitality you feel. Grains are not original human foods and nowadays many health challenges have been connected to them. I hope these recipes help you with transitioning to a more natural lifestyle if you have not already stopped eating grains. Please use them as long as you enjoy them or with friends and family and then feel free to leave them behind later. When you start to eat predominantly raw plant foods your taste buds naturally change.

Savoury Kamut Bread

250g kamut grain, soaked overnight to make about 375g (kamut is an older version of wheat - use spelt if kamut unavailable)
5 medium tomatoes
Salt and pepper
Fresh or dried herbs to taste – rosemary, oregano, basil, parsley, thyme etc
3 Sun-dried tomatoes, soaked in water for an hour plus soak water
A handful pumpkin seeds
2 Tbsps olive oil
2 sticks celery
optional:
Sprinkling Mushroom powders – cordyceps, lion's mane and tremella are my favourites (highly recommended)
½ bulb Fennel
½ cup flax seeds, ground
Process all the ingredients except the flax seeds together, adding water so that the mixture is quite soft.

Then add the flax seeds and process them in.
Spread into a layer about ¼ inch thick and sun dry or dehydrate in a dehydrator at 115 degrees until set.

We like this warm and soft with goat's butter and/or raw cheese

other extras:
1/8 onion
curry spices to taste
clove or two garlic

Flax Crackers

1 litre flax seeds
1 litre water
4 large tomatoes
1 red bell pepper
Juice of 1 lemon
Handful of Provencal herbs such as thyme, rosemary, basil
salt and pepper to taste
optional:
6 Tbsps unpasteurised miso

Soak flax seeds in the water for ½ hour.
Blend remaining ingredients.
Stir flax in.
Spread thinly on dehydrator trays
Dehydrate until crispy.
Store in airtight container.

This standard recipe can be varied by adding extra vegetables and seasonings such as miso.

Pizza with bread base

Bread Base

Use the Savoury Kamut Bread recipe.

Tomato Topping

2 tomatoes
4 halves sun-dried tomatoes, soaked

½ bell pepper
Optional: sprinkling dried basil and oregano
A little tomato soak water as necessary

Blend and spread on base.

Mushrooms

250g chestnut or other mushrooms, sliced
½ teaspoon Himalayan salt or sea salt
2 tablespoons olive oil
sprinkling lemon juice
Mix and dehydrate for 30 minutes

Other toppings

2 avocados, sliced
60g unpasteurised cheese, grated
12 olives, halved
Orange or yellow bell pepper, diced

Pumpkin Seed Pizza
Base:

500ml pumpkin seeds ,soaked
100g almonds or sunflower seeds, soaked
4 halves sun-dried tomatoes, soaked
½ tsp grated ginger
A drop chilli oil
Dash lemon juice

Process all these ingredients together until smooth and press out to form base.

Tomato Topping:

2 tomatoes
4 halves sun-dried tomatoes, soaked
½ bell pepper
Optional: sprinkling dried basil and oregano
A little tomato soak water as necessary

Blend and spread on base.

Other toppings:

2 avocados soaked
60g unpasteurised cheese, grated
12 olives, halved
orange or yellow bell pepper, diced

Serves 6

Buckwheat Pizza

Base:

500g buckwheat, soaked and sprouted
375ml flax seeds, soaked for ½ hour
375ml water
120ml olive oil
2 Tbsps dried basil
2 Tbsps dried oregano

Blend all ingredients except flax together.
Mix in flax
Shape into 1cm thick rounds on dehydrator sheets and dehydrate for until set

Tomato Sauce

5 large tomatoes
4 sun-dried tomatoes
1 shallot
½ Tbsp oregano
½ Tbsp basil

Blend until smooth

Other Toppings:

3 avocados, sliced
1 orange/yellow pepper, diced
a handful kalamata olives, pitted
100g raw cheese grated or sliced (choose an easy melting variety, varieties of Gruyère for example

Top pizza bases with tomato sauce and these toppings

Savoury Snacks

Dried Green Superfoods

In spring you can collect large quantities of wild greens and dry out in the dehydrator. To dry wild edible greens make sure any unknown plant material and debris is cleaned off. Spread evenly on dehydrator trays. Make sure they are thoroughly dry then crumble them with clean hands and store in airtight bags for the year ahead. You can potentially save a fortune on green superfoods this way, not to mention the satisfaction.

Make sure you know which greens are edible as there are some very poisonous ones around. Ideally take walk with a wild food expert in your area, failing that consult one of the many books now available.

Our favourites where we live in Devon include wild garlic leaves and flowers, violet flowers, pennywort, yellow archangel, cleavers, hawthorn leaves, bramble buds, gorse flowers, borage flowers, dandelion leaves and flowers, garlic mustard, crow garlic, rose garlic, nettles and dead nettles

If you dehydrate edible wild green leaves for a few hours and sprinkle on Himalayan salt and cold pressed olive oil they taste like crisps...a very moreish and mineral rich snack.

Spicy Nuts

250g almonds or walnuts, soaked overnight
1 or more teaspoons Hot Curry Powder to taste
sprinkling sea salt to taste (try ½ tsp as a starting point)
2 tsp olive oil

Mix all the ingredients and spread over a dehydrator tray.
Dehydrate until dry.
Store in an airtight box in a cool place

Desserts, Cakes, Puddings and Pies

The richer recipes here, especially those including nuts and dates are designed as invaluable special treats, in place of where you might have eaten problematic fats or sugars. They are great to share with friends and family and also as transition foods.. Day to day you probably are going to want eat to eat more of the simple smoothies and blends, especially long term. You can substitute dried fruits such as apricots and prunes for dates for less intense fruit sugar. Another substitution is lucuma powder with cacao butter to hold it together. This combination is spelled out in some of the raw cake recipes

Almond and Coconut Slice

Cake:

250g almonds, soaked overnight
4 ½ medjool dates
a handful coconut flakes, shredded coconut or fresh coconut
40g dried goji berries and/or 60g dried Montmorency cherries

Chocolate Topping:

60g cacao butter
30g lucuma
5g raw chocolate powder

Optional but amazing:
1g blue manna (for brain power)
1g he shou wu powder (for happy mood)
1g rosehip powder (for vitamin C and to bring out the flavour)

a few grains ground Himalayan salt or sea salt (helps with absorption of minerals and brings out flavour).
3g vanilla powder (for relaxation and flavour)
5g purple corn powder (for texture and brain chemicals)

Process almonds, coconut and dates together until smooth. A high quality processor like a Magi-mix is ideal here for a fluffy smoothness but any processor will work.
Add gojis and/or cherries to the mix and process until they are broken up.
Shape the mixture into a cake shape on a plate.
Melt cacao butter
Stir in other topping ingredients
Pour over the cake.
Cut into 12 slices.

Although raw food is generally nicest fresh, this cake is also lovely the next day when the goji berries have become soft like cherries and the flavours have mingled.

Hazelnut and Orange Slice

Cake:

125g almonds, soaked overnight
125g hazelnuts, soaked overnight
zest of 1 organic orange
4 ½ medjool dates

Chocolate Topping:

75g cacao butter

20g dried mulberries
1 tablespoon dried grated orange peel/zest
16g lucuma
3g raw cacao or cocoa powder
3g he shou wu
8g vanilla powder
dash cinnamon, allspice and ginger

Process almonds, hazelnuts, orange zest and dates together until smooth and fluffy.
Shape the mixture into a cake shape on a plate.

Melt cacao butter.
Stir in other topping ingredients.

Pour over the cake.
Cut into 12 slices.

Strawberry and Mango Tart

Base:
200g almonds, soaked
3 medjool dates

Topping:
400g strawberries
40g dried mango, soaked
2 medjool dates

Process the almonds and 3 dates and make into a pie base or several small tart bases.
Blend the remaining ingredients to make the topping.

It will set if given enough time – putting it in the fridge speeds this up.

Strawberry Cream Pie

Base:
250g almonds, soaked
4 medjool dates
½ tsp ground cinnamon

Topping:
1 punnet (about 300g) strawberries
flesh of 2 young coconuts or 1 mature coconut plus the juice
½ Tbsp lemon juice
3 medjool dates
¼ tsp ground cinnamon

Process the base ingredients and press into pie base shape.
Blend topping ingredients and spread over

Strawberry Pie

1 pint soaked almonds
10 medjool dates
1 kg strawberries
6 soaked dates with 60ml soak water
4 tsp psyllium husks

Combine almonds and dates together in a food processor to make pie base
Slice 2/3 of the strawberries and spread over the base
Blend the remaining strawberries with the dates and soak water and psyllium and use to cover the strawberries. This will set after a while.

Pear Crumble

150g almonds, soaked for a few hours or overnight
3 medjool dates
3 pears

Chop the pears up and put in the bottom of a dish
Process the almonds and dates until smooth and crumble over the pears.

Pears go particularly well but you can use any fruit for this recipe . Good combinations include apples, blackberries, apple and blackberry, apples and raisins, strawberries, and cherries.

Serve with kefir, live yogurt or raw crème fraiche.

Lemon Cheesecake

Base:

6 oz or 180g almonds, soaked overnight (makes about 1 pint)
4 medjool dates, pitted

Topping:

3 large bananas
3 large avocados
½ lemon

Process base ingredients together and press into a pie dish

Grate zest off lemon and squeeze out the juice.

Blend topping ingredients together and spread onto base.

Cherry Cheesecake

Base:
300g almonds, soaked
4 medjool dates

Cheese Layer:

8 dried apricots, soaked overnight
about 400g soft cheese. This can be kefir cheese, cream cheese or unseasoned cottage cheese made with 1200ml/2 pints milk
½ lemon – the zest and the juice

OR (non-dairy version)

4 large bananas
4 large avocados
½ lemon – the zest and the juice

Cherry Topping:

750g cherries, pitted
3 large or 5 small medjool dates, pitted
60ml water
4 teaspoons psyllium husks

Process the base ingredients and press into a 20cm round
Blend the cheese topping ingredients and spread over base
Spread 500g of the cherries on top of this.

Process the remaining 250g cherries,,dates and water until well mixed then add psyllium husks.
Spread this mixture over the cheese layer.

Black Forest Gateau
Cake:
500g carrots
2 bananas
150g pecans, preferably soaked and dehydrated
4 teaspoons raw chocolate (cacao) powder

Process the pecans until the texture of coarse flour.
Juice the carrots and put aside the juice for drinking or other recipes.
Mash the carrot pulp, bananas, pecans and cacao powder together until smooth and well mixed.

Buttercream:
6 medjool dates
1 ½ teaspoons raw chocolate power
4 or more tablespoons raw milk

Mash these ingredients together until smooth, adding the milk as necessary.

Cream:
5 tablespoons kefir cheese, raw crème fraiche or live yoghurt.

Cherry Filling:
300g cherries, chopped into quarters

'Kirsch':
3 tablespoons fermented fig water

(Soak a few, say 4, dried figs in just enough spring water to cover them for 24 hours. Use the surplus water as fig cordial)

Carob powder can be substituted for the raw chocolate powder in this recipe if you prefer.

Build up layers of gateau as follows:

1. One third of the cake mixture, spread into a round
2. half of the cream
3. one third of the cherries
4. one third of the cake mixture
5. kirsch sprinkled on
6. half the buttercream
7. one third of the cherries
8. last third of the cake
9. last half of the buttercream
10. last half of the cream
11. last third of the cherries

Black Forest Torte

A simpler version of Black Forest Gateau with the same components.

Spread the entire cake mixture on a dish.
Put a thick ring of the buttercream around the edge.
Fill the middle with the cream.
Place the cherries on top.

Non-dairy Version of Black Forest Gateau/Torte

Make substitutions as follows:

Buttercream:
Use hemp milk or almond milk rather than dairy milk.

Cream:
Blend 3 bananas and 3 tablespoons tahini together.

Banoffie Pie

Base:
250g almonds, soaked
3 medjool dates
¼ tsp ground cinnamon

Middle:
1 ½ bananas, sliced

Topping:
2 ½ bananas
2 medjool dates
eighth tsp cinnamon
small piece vanilla pod/ ¼ tsp vanilla powder (optional)
140g raw cashew nuts

Process the base ingredients and press into a pie base shape
Spread the sliced bananas over the base
Blend the topping ingredients until smooth and spread on top.

Pecan Pie

Base:

250g almonds, soaked
5 medjool dates or 200g lucuma combined with 12 Tablespoons cacao butter melted

Topping:

½ pint/250ml chopped avocado
½ pint/250ml soaked dates
1 lemon, squeezed
125g soaked pecans

Decoration:
50g pecans, soaked

Dry the 50g soaked pecans in a dehydrator until fairly crisp.
Process base ingredients and press into a pie dish.
Process the avocado, dates, lemon and 125g pecans and spread over base.
Decorate with the dried pecans.
Dehydrate the whole pie an hour or two until firm.

This recipe involves a bit of messing about with a dehydrator but is well worth it as it gives the pecans that special scrumptious flavour that they usually only have cooked. This is a lovely rich cooked tasting dessert. Pints is an unusual way to measure chopped fruit but it's quite simple – you just pile the chopped ingredient into the jug until it reaches the measure.

Butterscotch Pudding
by Bertie Whelan

¼ pint or 150ml raw milk or seed/nut milk
10 dried baby figs
3 dates
4 apricots
¼ oz or 10g butter/coconut butter (optional but delicious)

Blend the ingredients together until creamy and smooth. If using a high speed blender such as a vitamix there is no need to soak the dried fruit, but if not it will blend more easily if the dried fruits are soaked first.

Butterscotch Pie

250g pecans
2 medjool dates
double quantity Butterscotch Pudding recipe

Soak the pecans for a few hours or overnight then dehydrate
Process until the texture of coarse flour the add the dates and process together
Press into a pie dish
Top with the pudding mixture

Berry Coco Dessert

1 or 2 young coconuts
1 Tbsp lucuma
¼ tsp vanilla
300g berries or cherries (they can be frozen)

Blend fruit, lucuma, vanilla, flesh of coconut and about half the juice. One coconut is sometimes enough; if there is not enough flesh to make the mix creamy enough then use a second one. They do vary.
Serve topped with raw cream, dairy or otherwise.

Strawberry and Mango Pudding

400g strawberries
1 Tbsp sun-dried sun dried noni powder
40g dried mango, soaked
1/4 tsp vanilla powder
1 Tbsp raw honey

Blend ingredients

Serve with kefir or cream and sprinkled with 1 Tbs lucuma powder. Served on top of dairy milk kefir it is said to taste like 'fruit corner'.

Lucuma/Sapote and strawberry smoothie

This is a recipe specially for if you are lucky enough to find yourself in a place where there are fresh lucuma or sapote fruits available. If not you can substitute lucuma powder as shown.

1 banana
2 fresh lucuma or sapote (or lucuma powder plus another banana)
juice of 2 or 3 oranges
1 tsp sin dried noni powder
pinch vanilla powder
about 50ml cream
large punnet strawberries

Blend together

Bramble Pie and Coconut Cream

Base:
250g almonds, soaked overnight
5 – 10 medjool dates (number depends on size of dates and how sweet you would like it)

Fruit Layer:
500g blackberries

Filling:
500g blackberries
4 teaspoons psyllium
2 medjool dates

Coconut Cream:
2 young coconuts

Process base ingredients together and use to line a pie dish.
Pile the blackberries on top.
Blend the filling ingredients together and pour over the blackberries.
This will set.

To make the coconut cream blend the flesh of the coconuts with enough of the coconut water to make a creamy consistency.

Carob Pie

Base:
250g walnuts or hazelnuts, soaked overnight

1 tablespoon sun-dried (raw) carob powder
4 pitted medjool dates

Topping:
500ml avocado flesh
500ml soaked dates with their soak water
125ml sun-dried (raw) carob powder
Juice plus a little of the zest of one orange

Process the base ingredients together and press into a pie dish.
Process or blend the topping ingredients together.
Spread topping on base.

Optional extras:

Top with 250g cherries, pitted and halved
Add some ground hazelnut

Cherry Bakewell
Base:

250g almonds, soaked overnight
5 large dates or 9 medjool dates, pitted

Topping:

750g cherries, pitted
3 large or 5 small medjool dates, pitted
60ml water
4 teaspoons psyllium husks

Process the base ingredients until they stick together and the mixture is smooth.
Press into pie dish.
Arrange 500g cherries on the base.
Process the remaining 250g cherries,,dates and water until well mixed then add psyllium husks.
Spread this mixture over the cherries.

Golden Cherry Cream Pie
Pastry

100g or ½ cup almonds, soaked
100g or ½ cup hazelnuts/ filberts, soaked and dehydrated if possible
5 dates, fresh if possible or medjool
5 prunes
1 banana
30g pitted dried cherries or goji berries if not available
handful cacao nibs

Topping

hemp milk made from 2 to 3 cup hemp seeds and the juice of 2 oranges plus water as necessary
a few pieces orange peel/zest
2 dried figs
½ banana
50g or ¼ cup macadamia nuts
30g or a handful goji berries

Decoration

handful fresh cherries

sprinkling raw chocolate powder

Process all the pastry ingredients except the cacao nibs together until smooth, mix in the nibs and form the pastry base on a plate.
Blend the topping ingredients together until smooth and fill the pie. It will set in a few minutes.
Sprinkle the raw chocolate powder on the top and decorate with halved cherries

Fruit and Nut Cake

250g almonds, soaked
2 dried figs
2 dried apricots
5 prunes
2 fresh or medjool dates
30g currants/golden sultanas
30g goji berries/cranberries/dried cherries

Optional:
orange peel/zest
a handful pumpkin seeds
a handful fresh coconut

Process all the ingredients together except currants and gojis/cranberries/cherries until quite smooth.
Add gojis/cranberries/cherries and process until mixed in.
Add currants and process further.
Make into a cake shape.

This is a very moist cake and feels like a proper fruit cake.

Lotus Petal Cake

2 batches Fruit and Nut Cake
Raspberry Frosting / Raspberry Jam
Golden Cream
About 4 tablespoons bee pollen

Optional:

A handful of yacon
Form the cake mix into a flower shape with a middle and petals.
Top the middle with Golden Cream and cover with bee pollen and yacon.
Cover the petals with Raspberry Frosting / Raspberry Jam.

Each person can pull off a petal and the middle gets shared.

Golden Cream

150ml raw milk / hemp milk
60g macadamia nuts
2 teaspoons flax oil
1 banana
orange peel / zest
1 dried fig
1 dried apricot
10g goji berries
Blend all the ingredients together.

Raspberry Frosting

450g raspberries

3 dates
100ml raw milk/ sweet hemp milk

Blend

Use for coating cakes or as a sauce with desserts

Raspberry Jam

125g raspberries
3 fresh dates

Mash together

Pumpkin Pie
Base:

500ml walnuts, soaked overnight
4 medjool dates

Optional:
1 tablespoon carob powder

Topping:

1 litre pumpkin flesh
250ml dates, soaked overnight
1 avocado
1 teaspoon fresh grated ginger
eighth teaspoon allspice
eighth teaspoon cinnamon

dash lemon juice

To measure ingredients in volume this way just pile them in a measuring jug.

Process the base ingredients and press into a flan dish
Blend the topping ingredients and spread on base

For that fresh from the oven sensation warm in a dehydrator or briefly in a very low oven. Or you can make the topping warm by blending sufficiently long in a high power blender.

This recipe was translated from a cooked recipe by substituting dates for sugar and avocado for eggs and cream and using the same flavourings.

Mincemeat

110g currants, half soaked in water and half unsoaked
2 apples
30g almonds, soaked overnight
1 tablespoon lemon juice
zest of ¼ lemon
1 tablespoon coconut oil
sixteenth teaspoon each nutmeg, cinnamon and allspice or to taste
juice of 1 orange
3 soaked dates

Process the almonds into small pieces then add remaining ingredients except for the unsoaked currants. Process until the consistency if a wet mincemeat mixture. Stir in remaining currants.

Currants are used in this recipe because they are easy to obtain without the oil coating that raisins often have.

Mince Pies

Mincemeat:
as above recipe

Pastry:

200g almonds, soaked
6 dates / 3 medjool dates

Form pastry into small rounds or use to line a dish and fill with the mincemeat.

Serve with mild kefir, yoghurt or 'Custard' (see recipe)

Strawberry Sponge Cake

Cake:
250g almonds, soaked
3 medjool dates
2 apples

Optional:
handful dried apple
handful dried montmorency cherries

Filling:
100g strawberries, mashed

Toppings:
100g cherries, pitted
one recipe Cherry Sauce
one recipe Chocolate Topping for cake
handful Chocolate Cherries – dried Montmorency cherries dipped in the chocolate topping and allowed to set

Process almonds together until smooth and sticky
Add apples then remaining ingredients

Make one layer, add strawberries, then cover with second layer add toppings – any combination is delicious, especially all four.

Chocolate Topping for Cake

60g cacao butter
30g lucuma
5g cacao powder

Optional special extras:

1g blue manna/ crystal manna
1g he shou wu powder
1g rosehip powder
sprinkling Himalayan salt
3g vanilla powder
5g purple corn powder

Chocolate Cherries

Dip dried Montmorency cherries in the Chocolate Topping Recipe and allow to set in a dish.

Cherry Pudding

200g almonds, soaked
10g flaked coconut
5 medjool dates, pitted or 70g lucuma and 4 Tbsps melted cacao butter to set the base
1 apple
30g dried Montmorency cherries

Process almonds, coconut and dates until mixture is sticky and holds together.
Slice the apple off the core and process in.
Add cherries and process until just a little broken down.

Serve with Cherry Sauce.

Coconut Cherry Cream Pie

Base:
300g Brazil nuts
100g lucuma and 6 Tbsps cacao butter to set the base

Topping:
300g cherries (frozen is fine)
flesh of 2 young coconuts
½ Tbsp lemon juice

3 medjool dates

Process the base ingredients and press into pie base shape.
Blend topping ingredients and spread over

Coconut CreamTopping (optional):
2 young coconuts

To make the coconut cream blend the flesh of the coconuts with enough of the coconut water to make a creamy consistency.

Sweet Sauces

Cherry Coulis

250g cherries or other red fruit such as strawberries, plums etc
50g dried Montmorency cherries
1 medjool date

Blend all the ingredients together until smooth.
This sauce sets in a while and can be used to top cheesecakes, cakes and other desserts or poured over ice-creams.

Coconut Cream
Coconut flesh
Coconut juice
optional: small piece of vanilla pod or sprinkling of vanilla powder

Blend until as smooth as possible

Young coconuts work best but fresh mature coconuts are fine too.

There is a knack to opening a mature coconut. There is a group of three hole marks at the top of the coconut – one of these is much softer than the others. You can make a hole through it with the points of closed scissors and pour the juice out. After that smash it open by throwing it hard onto a concrete path or hitting it with a hammer. You can then prise the coconut flesh out.

Three Different Ways to make a Custard Substitute

Custard 1

2 custard apples (cherimoyas)
2 avocados, peeled and stoned

Take seeds out of the custard apples (you really need to get into the flesh with your fingers) and blend with the avocados.
This is caramelly and very like traditional custard.

Custard 2

2 bananas, peeled
2 avocados, peeled and stoned

Simply blend together. This makes a very fine second best to Custard 1 if, as is usually the case, custard apples are not available. It makes a nice mousse in its own right.

Custard 3
1 banana

1 avocado
2 ½ oz or 75ml milk
5 dried baby figs
2 dates
2 apricots

Blend all the ingredients together until smooth and creamy. This is quite like a caramel custard too and the small amount of milk is a satisfying touch.

Strawberry Jelly

250g strawberries (can be frozen)
½ cup chia seeds soaked in equal amount of water
3 bananas
4 cups coconut
Blend all the ingredients.
Refrigerate for a few hours until set.

Ice-creams

Raw ice cream can be made very easily and, because of the consistency of raw fruits you don't even need an ice-cream maker. You simply blend a combination of fresh fruit and frozen fruit and other raw ingredients to taste, using a sturdy blender.
Another option is to put it all through a twin gear juicer.
 After that it can be eaten or if you prefer it firmer you can freeze it in ice cube containers or a tub. If using an ice-cream maker just pour the blended mixture in and let it do its thing. In that case you do not need to freeze any of the fruit beforehand although of you do it will speed the process up.

Ice Cream Cones

Blend any mixture of fruit and spread on dehydrator sheets and dry until set but still pliable.

Cut into shapes and wrap into cone shapes to contain Ice-cream.
This is a great way of using up left over scraps of fruit. The pieces can also be used as a fruit snack.

Banana and Sesame Ice cream

4 banana, frozen without their skins
1 fresh banana
60ml sesame seeds, ground
¼ vanilla pod
1 tablespoon coconut oil

Put unfrozen banana in bottom of blender jug and add other ingredients
Blend until smooth then serve immediately.
This recipe really needs a sturdy blender.

An alternative way of making this ice-cream is to mix the ingredients together and put through a heavy duty cog-based juicer.

Blackberry Ice-cream

2 punnets blackberries
1 recipe Chocolate Pudding, frozen
3 fresh bananas

Blend.

A sturdy blender is needed for this recipe and the best results are achieved in a high power blender even better results put through an ice-cream maker.

Serves 4 - 6

Blackberry Sorbet

4 frozen bananas
2 fresh bananas
1 punnet blackberries

Blend
For even better results put through an ice-cream maker.

serves 4

Cherry Ice Cream

2 fresh bananas
2 frozen peeled bananas
125g frozen cherries
15g dried montmorency cherries

optional:
 a little vanilla pod or powder

Note: remove the skins before freezing the bananas and break them up into pieces. Pit the cherries before freezing them too.

Blend all the ingredients together.

Serve with cherry sauce

Because of the abundance of melatonin in montmorency cherries, this is a great evening dessert especially for young children when you want to settle them early.

Lemon Ice Cream

2 bananas
2 frozen peeled bananas
zest and juice of 1 lemon.

Blend all the ingredients together.

Choc Mint Ice Cream

2 bananas
2 frozen peeled bananas
a few mint or peppermint leaves
a handful of cacao nibs

Blend the bananas and leaves.
Stir in cacao nibs.

Chocolate Hemp Ice Cream

Make a batch of the Chocolate Pudding in the Breakfast section including hemp leaf powder and freeze for a few hours.

Sweet Treats

Hazelnut Truffles

15g hazelnuts, soaked and dehydrated
15g goji berries
30g fresh coconut
20g raw cacao nibs
2g vanilla powder

grind ingredients together – this is easiest in the type of grinder attachment that you turn upside down onto a blender
shape into balls

optional extras:
for extra sweetness:
1 dried fig/10g lucuma

for extra nutrition:
5g maca
3g mesquite

for extra nice feeling/taste:
dash he shou wu
crystal manna
5g cacao powder
a little orange zest

to set better:
10g cacao butter, melted
mix in after grinding

chocolate topping:
can coat with chocolate:
30g cacao butter
15g lucuma
5g cacao powder
10g raw milk
dash of vanilla powder

cherry truffles:
shape balls round fresh cherries or dried Montmorency cherries
(chocolate and cherries go together so well)

Fig Balls
by Lizzy Paige

9 dates
15 apricots
5 dried figs
2 Tbsp coconut butter

Combine in a sturdy food processor and roll the sticky mixture into balls.

Alternative recipe:

10 large dried figs
5 dried apricots
3 dates
1 Tbsp coconut butter
flaked coconut

Whir all the ingredients up then when you're finished roll them up and put them in a bowl.

Whir up some flaked coconut until fine.
Combine in a sturdy food processor and roll the sticky mixture into balls
Roll the balls in the coconut.

Almond Balls

250g almonds, soaked
2 dried figs
2 dried apricots
5 prunes
2 fresh dates
30g currants
30g goji berries
Optional: orange peel/zest

Sprinklings of any selection of the following superfoods:

vanilla powder
he shou wu
suma
rosehip
maca
raw chocolate powder

Optional:
a few chunks fresh coconut

Process all the ingredients together except currants until quite smooth.
Add currants and process further.
Shape into balls.

Jungle Bars

100g wild jungle peanuts
80g dried mulberries
Process together until sticky. (If necessary add a tiny bit of water to make this happen.)
Shape into four bars or balls

Basic Raw Chocolate Recipe

60g cacao butter, melted
30g lucuma
10g raw cacao powder

Holly's Raw Chocolate

60g cacao butter
30g lucuma
5g raw chocolate powder
Optional but delicious and energising:
1g blue manna/3g crystal manna
1g he shou wu powder
1g rosehip powder
sprinkling Himalayan salt
3g vanilla powder
5g purple corn powder

Melt the cacao butter in a dehydrator or in small bowl resting in a larger container of hot water.
Stir in the rest of the ingredients.
Pour into chocolate moulds or pretty ice cube moulds

Super Magical Fruit Raw Chocolate

60g cacao butter
40g cacao paste
3 Tbsps raw honey
a few grains Celtic sea salt
sprinkling cayenne powder

2 Tbsps maca powder (gelatinised maca works best)
3 Tbsps lucuma powder
2 Tbsps violet or green fig powder
1 Tbsp acerola cherry powder/strawberry powder
½ tsp vanilla powder
1 Tbsp purple corn flour
1 Tbsp hemp leaf powder
1 tsp he shou wu powder

Optional:
1 Tbsp raw carob powder
1 tsp algarroba/mesquite
sprinkling blue green algae
1 Tbsp raw noni powder (slightly alters taste)
mucuna
a few drops peppermint essence

For milk chocolate: add powdered raw colostrum

Strawberry Milk Chocolate

50g cacao butter
25g lucuma
5g chocolate powder

6 strawberries, chopped up
20 ml raw milk

Melt cacao butter in a dehydrator or in a bowl over another bowl of hot water.
Stir in lucuma and chocolate powder.
Beat in milk then stir in strawberries.
Put into a bowl to set.

Honey Chocolate

100g cacao butter, melted
4tbs raw chocolate powder
3 Tbsps lucuma
2 Tbsps mesquite
3 Tbsps honey

Mix all the ingredients and pour into moulds and let set.

Lucuma Fudge

100g cacao butter
3 tablespoons lucuma
3 tablespoons maca
2 tablespoons mesquite
2 tablespoons raw cold-pressed honey

Melt cacao butter over warm water. Mix in other ingredients and pour into chocolate moulds to set.

Festive Chocolate

75g cacao butter
20g dried mulberries
1 tablespoon grated orange zest, dried (in dehydrator is easy way)
16g lucuma
3g cacao seed powder
3g he shou wu
8g vanilla powder
dash cinnamon, allspice and ginger

Melt cacao butter in dehydrator or over a bowl of warm water
Grind mulberries and orange zest together in coffee grinder
Mix all ingredients together and pour into chocolate moulds or ice cube trays and set in fridge or freeze

Raw Chocolate Biscuits

400g Brazil nuts
100g lucuma
60g cacao butter
1 recipe Supermagical Fruit Raw Chocolate

Melt cacao butter
Process Brazils and Lucuma
Mix in cacao butter.

Grease plate/dish with coconut butter.
Press the mixture into it
Top with chocolate.

Simple Yoghurt, Cheese and Kefir Making

Yoghurt

Warm raw milk gently in a saucepan stirring all the while until body temperature (37°- you can test with a finger), stir in a couple of dessert spoonfuls natural live yoghurt. Rinse a glass lined vacuum flask with hot water, pour in the milk and yoghurt mixture, seal up and leave overnight. In the morning you will have delicious fresh warm yoghurt to eat.

My first experience of eating warm yoghurt in the morning was many years ago in Sri Lanka - a very different experience to eating it out of a tub from the fridge!

Greek Yoghurt

If you use Greek-style live yoghurt as a starter you get a delicious creamy yoghurt – the culture is slightly different. You can get it even thicker buy putting a small amount Greek yoghurt in milk in a glass bowl in a dehydrator overnight. Just be careful not to break the bottom of the dehydrator with the weight.

Cream cheese

Allow Greek style yoghurt to strain through muslin until the liquid has drained off.

Cottage Cheese

Warm a pint of raw milk (goat's, cow's or sheep's), taking care not to heat above body temperature (37°C) then added a little mesophilic starter and leave for an hour. Then re-warm it and added 20 drops of vegetarian rennet.

This can then set in less than an hour when the whey is strained off by tipping it into a muslin cloth over a bowl. If using in a cheesecake then add no further ingredients but as a savoury you can add ground sea salt to bring out the flavour and other ingredients such as dried garlic leaves and chives, sun-dried tomatoes, and different herbs.
For details about where to obtain cheese starters see list of suppliers at back of book. You can buy rennet from health food stores.

This cheese, seasoned with salt and pepper is lovely with raw sprouted breads such as Savoury Kamut Bread.

Kefir

Milk kefir and water kefir are two different kinds of SCOBY (symbiotic culture of yeast and bacteria). Milk kefir needs to be fed a raw animal milk on a long term basis in order to thrive, whilst water kefir needs a sugar solution such as sugar water, fruit juice or coconut water.

Kefir – the Magic Elixir
(milk kefir)

Kefir is a culture which I described earlier as a number one magical food. I have seen so many benefits to people over the years who are equally enchanted by the mystery of it's origins, I have created many recipes using it.

Kefir is very easy to make. You need to obtain a starter culture which can be done on-line. You just put the culture into the raw milk in an airtight glass jar (a kilner jar is ideal). The process is anaerobic (happens better without oxygen). Metal can damage kefir if it touches it. Plastic is no good for any period of time as the kefir, being acidic will slightly corrode the plastic into the kefir. Just leave at room temperature for about 24 hours, strain with a plastic sieve and use the liquid that drains out for eating, drinking or recipes. Store the liquid in the fridge until you use it. You can rinse the kefir culture itself (the lumpy bits) with lukewarm water but traditionally this was not done and this may have preserved the integrity of the grains better. Wash the jar with hot water and put them back into the clean jar. Kefir is anti-bacterial – there is no need for any special sterilising solutions just common sense hygiene.

Raw milk is preferable but not essential for making kefir and cows', goats', and sheep's milk are all suitable. If you cannot find unpasteurised milk then one of the benefits of kefir is that it will put a lot of life-force and structure back into the milk. We only make kefir with animal milks and are happy to make it this way but it is made by some people with non-animal milks such as soy, coconut, nut or seed milks. Fruit needs to be added to these milks to give the culture the sugars it needs.

Kefir is a living thing, can live forever and can be used indefinitely. If kept at room temperature it will continue to grow (doubling in size about every 16 days) and the extra culture can given away or even eaten.

If not making kefir for a while, store the culture in a mixture of water and milk in the fridge. Store spare culture in this way until you find someone else who wants it.

Kefir is lovely poured over crumbles or chocolate pudding or blended into spicy savoury sauces.

Full Kefir Instructions for References Purposes

Kefir can be made from almost any kind of milk – cows', goat's, sheep's, soy, coconut, nut milks and seed milks – but not rice or oat milk as they are quite different. I have made delicious kefir from unpasteurised cow's milk (biodynamic Jersey cow's milk is particularly nice and creamy) and raw goat's milk. Non-animal milk may need to be sweetened for example with soaked dried fruit blended in. Many people use coconut milk with success. The kefir culture grows better if fed some animal milk from time to time. You may wish to try making kefir from any milk you choose, depending on how you feel about these things, how your body reacts and what is locally available to you.

You just put the culture into the raw milk in an airtight glass jar (a kilner jar is ideal). The process is anaerobic (happens better without oxygen). Metal can damage kefir if it touches it. Plastic is no good for any period of time as the kefir, being acidic will slightly corrode the plastic into the kefir. Just leave at room temperature for about 24 hours, strain with a nylon sieve and use the liquid that drains out for eating, drinking or recipes. Store the liquid in the fridge until you use it. Clean the jar with hot water and put the lumpy bits (culture) back into the jar. You can rinse the lumpy bits with lukewarm water before you return them to the jar but traditionally they were not washed and this may be better for them.

If not making kefir for a while store the culture in a mixture of water and milk in the fridge. Kefir culture multiplies very quickly – store spare culture in this way until you find someone else who wants it. You can also dehydrate at lowest temperature available in a dehydrator. It takes many hours for the kefir grains to completely dry out. When they do they are golden colour. They are best kept cool if storm for a period of time but you can travel with them and this is a useful option for transporting them over long distances.

To reactivate dehydrated kefir grains, choose a safe spot at room temperature and out of direct sunlight, also away from a rubbish or compost bin or any other cultured foods. Cross-contamination by stray yeasts and bacteria can be problematic for the kefir grains. Place the dehydrated kefir grain in one cup of fresh milk, preferably raw and leave in a partially sealed glass container such as kilner jar at room temperature. The kefir thrives in this kind of container also it protects it from unwanted pests. After about 24 hours strain the grains with a nylon sieve and add to fresh milk. You do this even if the milk does not thicken. The strained milk can be discarded or consumed provided it looks and smells okay. Repeat this process daily. Within 4-7 days, the 24-hour milk batch will begin to smell sour but clean. Eventually the milk will start to coagulate the milk will turn into kefir liquid within 24-hours. During the first few days you may see an overgrowth of yeast or a layer or froth or foam on the surface of the milk. Within 5-7 days, the bacterial balance should stabilise and the kefir will begin to smell clean and sour. Under some circumstances, the kefir grains may take 2-4 weeks to start to making kefir. Once the milk is reliably turning to pleasant tasting and pleasant smelling kefir within 24-48 hours, your kefir grains are ready to generate regular batches of kefir and you can follow the instructions provided onto how to make kefir.

Signs of problems during rehydration are helpful to know. These problems are relatively uncommon, but it is important to keep an eye out for these few signs that the process isn't proceeding normally. If the milk is changed every 24 hours for more than 10 days and the milk is not turning to kefir within 24 hours, allow the milk and kefir grains to sit for an additional 24 hours (48 hours total). Ambient temperature in particular can affect how quickly the kefir forms. If the milk still fails to coagulate contact us to determine if the culture is inactive and if a replacement is needed. While unusual, mould can and does occasionally develop and can generally be seen by the formation of white, green, orange, red, or black spots on the surface of the milk. If mould does develop, immediately throw away the entire batch including the kefir grains.

Coconut Kefir
('water kefir')

As described earlier water kefir, also known as Tibiscos, is a different scoby to milk kefir. It is a great alternative for those who do not wish to drink milk kefir as it is also a probiotic. It needs to be fed liquids containing sugar such as sugar water, fruit juice, or coconut water. Some people use fructose water or fruit blended with water. Coconut juice/water is our favourite. It's simple and clean. You can purchase both kinds of cultures in many places nowadays including online. Coconut water kefir is a delicious drink and is also useful as an inoculant for making fermented vegetables, protecting the fermentation process from unwanted outside bacteria. Lactobacilli are on the cabbage already but adding coconut kefir increases the diversity of the bacteria and acts to protect the fermentation process. You can make many different recipes by adding fruit or fruit juices. Be aware water kefir is very slightly alcoholic, in a similar manner to kombucha, and generally more so than milk kefir, so is best drunk in moderation.

Recipes made with Kefir

Kefir Cheese

If you can get the kefir thick enough, it can be made into cheese. Simply pour into a muslin bag (I use the bags that I use for making hemp milk) and hang over a container to catch the whey. Leave for 24 hours and you have kefir cheese in the bag.

Vanilla Kefir Elixir

250ml (½ pint milk) kefir
½ tsp vanilla powder
2 Tbsps lucuma powder

Mix ingredients together for a sweet fizzy yoghurty drink.

Chocolate Kefir Cheesecake

Be aware that the kefir cream cheese needs to be prepared at least one day in advance.
Base ingredients:
200g Brazil nuts
100g macadamia nuts
4 – 5 medjool dates or 100g lucuma and 6 Tablespoons cacao butter

Chocolate ingredients:
4oz or 110g cacao butter
2oz or 60g cacao paste
3 Tbsps raw honey or yacon syrup
pinch cayenne
pinch Celtic sea salt
3 Tbsps lucuma powder
2 Tbsp maca
1 tsp he shou wu
1 Tbsp strawberry powder
1 Tbsp fig powder
1 Tbsp purple corn powder

¼ tsp vanilla powder
¼ tsp blue green algae

Cheese ingredients:
300g kefir cream cheese
Kefir cream cheese can be made in one of two ways:
1. Pour kefir into a muslin bag and put in a nylon sieve over a bowl to catch the whey. Leave for 24 hours and you have kefir cheese in the bag.
2. Leave kefir in a jar until it separates into curds and whey. This take a few days. Then you scoop the curd off the top as your kefir cream cheese.

To make base:
Process nuts and dates and spread on pie plate.
To make chocolate:
Melt cacao paste and butter over hot water, add honey and salt Mix dry chocolate ingredients

To make the cheesecake:
Stir the molten chocolate into the cream cheese thoroughly and spread on base.
You can put a layer of kefir cream cheese underneath the chocolate layer or spread on top of it, then sprinkle with cacao powder, vanilla powder, blue green algae etc as in the picture.

Cherry Chocolate Kefir Cheesecake

Base:

200g brazils
100g macadamias
4 medjool dates or substitute about 100g lucuma and 6 Tbsps cacao butter to set the base

Chocolate ingredients:
110g cacao butter
50g cacao paste
3 Tbsps honey or yacon syrup
inch cayenne
pinch sea salt
4 Tbsps lucuma powder
1 Tbsp maca
1 tsp he shou wu
1 Tbsp strawberry powder
1 Tbsp fig powder
1 Tbsp purple corn
1/4 tsp vanilla powder
1/4 teaspoon blue green algae optional
1 Tbsp hemp leaf powder
300g kefir cream cheese

Process nuts and dates or lucuma and cacao butter and spread on pie plate
Melt cacao paste and butter over hot water, add honey/yacon and salt
Mix dry chocolate ingredients
Stir paste and butter mixture into dry ingredients
Then stir the molten chocolate into the cream cheese thoroughly and spread on base.
You can put a layer of kefir cream cheese underneath the chocolate layer also a strawberry cream cheese layer.
You could also make a second batch of chocolate as fourth layer
You could also top with cherry coulis
Berry cream cheese layer:
big punnet strawberries / frozen berries
kefir cheese made from 1 litre milk
2 Tbsps honey
100g cacao butter to set

Cherry Coulis:
250g cherries or other red fruit such as strawberries, plums etc
50g dried montmorency cherries
1 medjool date

Blend all the ingredients together until smooth.

Cherry/Berry Cream
1 – 2 young coconuts
300g berries/cherries - can be frozen
1 Tbsp lucuma
1 Tbsp honey
1/4 tsp vanilla
300g berries/cherries - can be frozen

Blend fruit, lucuma, vanilla, flesh of coconut and about half the juice. 1 coconut may be enough; if there is not enough flesh to make the mix creamy enough then use a second one.

Pear and Pecan Cheesecake

125g pecan nuts
1 pear, grated
200g kefir cheese/cream cheese/unseasoned cottage cheese made with 1 pint or 600ml milk
2 medjool dates

Soak the pecans overnight and then dry them for a few hours, ideally in a dehydrator or in warm sunshine. This gives them a flavour similar to cooked pecans.

Process the pecans until they look like coarse flour and then mix with the grated pear. Press onto a dish to make the base.

Mash the medjool dates into the kefir cheese and spread onto the base.

Chocolate Kefir

2Tbsp raw chocolate powder
8 fresh or medjool dates
250ml mild kefir

Mash dates.
Add chocolate powder and kefir gradually.

Lasagna Deluxe

Creamy Pasta Sauce:

2 large tomatoes
1 red/orange/yellow pepper
6 tablespoons kefir cheese or other soft mild unpasteurised cheese
4 sun-dried tomatoes, soaked
2 teaspoons hemp oil
Blend all the ingredients together until smooth and creamy

'Pasta'

1 courgette

Slice very thinly. The best results are with a potato peeler.

Green layer:

About 250g mixed greens, wild or fresh salad leaves

1 cucumber
3 sticks celery
2 sun-dried tomatoes
1 avocado
1 Tbsp coriander
A little chilli
3 small carrots
1 pepper
2 tomatoes
1 floret broccoli
25g currants
A little dulse
About ½ Tbsp each:
Cinnamon
Lemongrass
Basil
Fennel seeds

Process all the ingredients together until broken down.

Cheese Sauce:

Hemp milk made with 225g hemp seeds, soaked
50g sunflower seeds, soaked
50g pumpkin seeds, soaked
25g walnuts, soaked
25g sesame seeds, soaked
75g Parmesan cheese
1 Tbsp flax oil
Blend all the ingredients together until smooth.

Grated Cheese topping:

25g parmesan cheese

Layer as follows:

1. ½ creamy pasta sauce
2. ½ courgette
3. ½ green layer
4. ½ cheese sauce
5. ½ creamy pasta sauce
6. ½ courgette
7. ½ green layer
8. ½ cheese sauce
9. grated parmesan

All this can be warmed – the sauces in a saucepan on low heat and the whole thing in an oven at low heat or in a dehydrator. Just make sure it doesn't go over body temperature.

Delicious served over a crisp green salad and grated cucumber

Cream of Watercress and Strawberry Soup

½ pint mild kefir
1 bunch watercress
a handful strawberries
dash of cayenne powder
1 tablespoon lucuma powder (optional)

Blend all ingredients together

Coconut Water Kefir

1 tablespoons or more water kefir grains
1 litre coconut Water

Place the water kefir grains in a kilner jar.
Add the coconut water
In a few days it will be bubbling while still slightly sweet, this is the time to drink it, use it or refrigerate it. You simply need to strain through a nylon sieve.

Kefir Coconut Ginger Beer

This is an example of the simplicity of coconut water recipes, you can make many different recipes adding fruit or fruit juices. Be aware water kefir is very slightly alcoholic, in a similar manner to kombucha, and is not for drinking regularly in large amounts.

up to 3 tablespoons water kefir grains
1 litre coconut Water
1 tsp grated Ginger

Place the water kefir grains in a kilner jar.
Add the coconut water and ginger
In a few days it will bubble while still slightly sweet, this is the time to drink it or refrigerate it. Strain through a nylon sieve.

Fermented Vegetables and Krauts

Golden Garden Vegetable Kraut

4 cabbages, white, green and red
2 carrots organic and preferably heirloom
1 small sweet potato
2 spring onions
2 roots/120g ginger root
2 garlic cloves
½ tablespoon rosehip powder (optional extra)
1 teaspoon sea salt
125ml coconut water kefir

Process or grate all vegetables, mix and put into 20 litre crock or several kilner jars
add the coconut kefir and 125ml spring water with sea salt
cover with whole cabbage leaves

Ferment about 10 days

Spicy Tomato Salsa

1 kg tomatoes, chopped
3 onions, chopped
1 chilli, seeds removed and chopped
1 clove garlic, minced
handful fresh coriander, chopped
1 lime, juiced
dash sea salt
about 50ml coconut kefir

1 cabbage leaf

Blend a third of the tomatoes and onion plus the chilli and garlic together.
Add the rest of the tomatoes, onion, and other ingredients, coriander, salt and lime juice.
Put into large kilner jar.
Cover with coconut kefir.
Cover with cabbage leaf to keep the mix under the water.
After a day or two it will start to bubble, taste it each day to test when it tastes good, probably after a few days depending on the exact conditions.

Asian Kimchee

6 cabbages
1 bunch carrots
1 chilli, chopped
250g dried arame or other seaweed, soaked until soft in warm water
3 teaspoons mushroom mycelium powders such as reishi, lion's mane, cordyceps, tremella, shitake
handful goji berries
small handful schizandra berries (optional)
3 teaspoons sea salt
¼ litre coconut kefir
¼ litre spring water

Process or grate cabbages and carrots.
Add seaweed, mushroom powders, goji berries and schizandra.
Mix and put into 10 litre crock or several kilner jars.
Add ½ litre coconut kefir and ½ litre spring water with sea salt
Cover with whole cabbage leaves
Ferment for about 5 - 10 days, depending on exact conditions, taste after a few days.

References, Reading and Resources

Here are books, papers and websites referenced in this book, further recommended reading, also resources and suppliers.

My websites:

www.foodforconsciousness.co.uk
www.edenicstates.com
www.hollyjrpaige.com
foodforconsciousness,blogspot.co.uk

Origins ~ Your Unique Codes for Life

Return to the Brain of Eden by Tony Wright and Graham Gynn
Quest for the Zodiac: The Cosmic Code Beyond Astrology by John Lash

What on Earth's going on ~ the Human Story

Return to the Brain of Eden by Tony Wright and Graham Gynn
Not in His Image by John Lash
Memories and Visions of Paradise: Exploring the Universal Myth of a Lost Golden Age by Richard Heinberg
Parzival by Wolfram von Eschenbach and A. Hatto
Food of the Gods by Terence McKenna
Voices of the First Day: Awakening in the Aboriginal Dreamtime Robert Lawlor
The Biology of Belief: Unleashing the Power of Consciousness, Matter & Miracles by Bruce H. Lipton

The Century of the Self, 2002 British television documentary series by Adam Curtis.
Hypernormalization, 2016 documentary by Adam Curtis
Forbidden Dimensions by C. G. Browne
Savant Syndrome: An Extraordinary Condition A Synopsis: Past, Present, Future by Darold A. Treffert, MD

Tony Wright's websites:
www.leftinthedark.org.uk
beyond-belief.org.uk
https://web.archive.org/web/20160205024447/http://beyond-belief.org.uk/

John Lash's websites:
metahistory.org
gaiaspora.org

Eating the Biological Diet of our Species

Neurogenesis by Brant Cortright
Conscious Eating by Gabriel Cousens
The Mood Cure by Julia Ross
Food for Free by Richard Mabey
Nutrition and Physical Degeneration by Weston A. Price
Dead Doctors Don't Lie Joel Wallach
Colloidal Minerals and Trace Elements How to Restore the Body's Natural Vitality Marie France Muller
Minerals for the Genetic Code Charles Walters
The Miraculous Results Of Extremely High Doses Of The Sunshine Hormone Vitamin D3; My Experiment With Huge Doses Of D3 From 25,000 To 50,000 To 100,000 Iu A Day Over A 1 Year Period by Jeff T. Bowles
Superfoods by David Wolfe

Raw Food Works by Diana Store , Gabriel Cousens, Brian R Clement
Mycelium Running: A Guide to Healing the Planet through Gardening with Gourmet and Medicinal Mushrooms by Paul Stamets
Superfoods for Optimal Health: chlorella and spirulina by Mike Adams
The Tooth Cure by Ramiel Nagel
Gut Reactions: How healthy insides can improve your weight, mood and well-being by Justin Sonnenburg (Author), Erica Sonnenburg
The Hidden Messages in Water by Masaru Emoto
'Cancer, Why were dying to know the truth' Phillip Day

Papers byKatherine Milton PhD :
Micronutrient intakes of wild primates: are humans different?
Back to Basics: Why Foods of Wild Primates have Relevance for Modern Human Health
Nutritional Characteristics of Wild Primate foods: Do the Diets of our Closest Living Relatives Have Lessons for Us

Online references for vitamin D:
Influence of season and latitude on the cutaneous synthesis of vitamin D3: exposure to winter sunlight in Boston and Edmonton will not promote vitamin D3 synthesis in human skin.
www.ncbi.nlm.nih.gov/pubmed/2839537
www.naturalnews.com/027345_Vitamin_D_sun_exposure_blood.html
www.naturalnews.com/028357_vitamin_D_deficiency.html
www.naturalnews.com/030500_vitamin_D_absorption.html

Websites about Weston Price's work:
westonaprice.org
ppnf.org

The Blue Zones Solution: Eating and Living Like the World's Healthiest People by Dan Buettner
Brain Maker: The Power of Gut Microbes to Heal and Protect Your Brain - for Life by David Perlmutter

Grain Brain: The Surprising Truth about Wheat, Carbs, and Sugar - Your Brain's Silent Killers by David Perlmutter
No Grain, No Pain by Peter Osbourne

Brain Biochemicals to Optimise Potential

The Melatonin Miracle: Nature's Age-Reversing, Disease-Fighting, Sex-Enhancing Hormone by Walter Pierpaoli
DMT The Spirit Molecule by Dr Rick Strassman
Iboga: The Visionary Root of African Shamanism by Vincent Ravalec and Mallendi
Ibogaine Explained by Peter Frank

Living in Beauty ~ Natural Lifestyle

Earthing: The Most Important Health Discovery Ever by Clinton Ober and Stephen T Sinatra
We Borrow the Earth by Patrick Jasper Lee
Coming Home to the Trees by Patrick Jasper Lee
Anastasia and The Ringing Cedars Series by Vladimir Megre
Plant Spirit Healing: A Guide to Working with Plant Consciousness by Pam Montgomery and Stephen Harrod Buhner
Biogenic Living by Edmond Bordeaux Szekely
Dr. Dietrich Klinghardt – called Smart Meters & EMR - The Health Crisis Of Our Time. www.youtube.com/watch?v=PktaaxPl7RIClint Ober on Earthing www.youtube.com/watch?v=lY3w8kDn2Eo Grounded (the documentary) www.youtube.com/watch?v=b8b_lg2z8Ncfindaspring.com

Cleansing and Regenerating your Body Ecology

The Body Ecology Diet: Recovering Your Health and Rebuilding Your Immunity Donna Gates

Kefir Rediscovered by Klaus Kaufmann
The Second Brain Michael D Gershon
The Amazing Liver and Gallbladder Flush Andreas Moritz
Niacin cleanse:
articles.mercola.com/sites/articles/archive/2014/05/04/detoxification-program.aspx
Gut and Psychology Syndrome www.gaps.me

Reclaiming and Sustaining your Mind

Forbidden Dimensions. Primitivism, Prehistory and the Posthuman Era by C G Browne
Tapping the Healer Within by Roger J Callahan
Why People Don't Heal and How they Can by Caroline Myss
Complaining is Terrible for you according to Science by Jessica Stillman. www.inc.com/jessica-stillman/complaining-rewires-your-brain-for-negativity-science-says.html
Imagining the Tenth Dimension: A New Way of Thinking About Time and Space by Rob Bryanton
Imagining the tenth dimension tenthdimension.com by Rob Bryanton
Free guide to tapping AT Roger Callahan's site at www.rogercallahan.com and www.thetappingsolution.com and a free guide to EFT at Gary Craig's site www.garythink.com.

Michael Flanagan on the Neurophone:
www.youtube.com/watch?v=bCRJeB_W9Ec
www.youtube.com/watch?v=yY__FEBjaXg
www.youtube.com/watch?v=r71StfcWjUM

The Manchester Trial , the study on sleep deprivation on raw diet www.leftinthedark.org.uk/PDF/THE%20MANCHESTER%20TRIAL.pdf
Strategic Intervention Handbook: How to quickly produce profound change in yourself and others by Magali Peysha and Mark Peysha

Mind intrusion www.metahistory.org/gnostique/archonfiles/AlienDreaming.php

Our Hormonal Human Life Cycle

The Continuum Concept by Jean Liedloff
Cupid's Poisoned Arrow: From Habit to Harmony in Sexual Relationships by Marnia Robinson
Venus on Fire, Mars on Ice: Hormonal Balance--The Key to Life, Love, and Energy by John Gray
Die Wise – A Manifesto for Sanity and Soul Stephen Jenkinson

Recent Secular Trends in Pubertal Timing http://www.karger.com/Article/Pdf/336325

'Melatonin increases oestrogen receptor binding activity.': www.nature.com/nature/journal/v305/n5932/abs/305323a0.html

Tony Wright explains how oestrogen dominance has led to reproductive problems and cancers and points out the benefits of flavonoids. beyond-belief.org.uk/sites/beyond-belief.org.uk/files/Copy%20of%20Oestrogen%20dependent%20cancer.pdf

Recipes

Raw Living by Kate Magic
Raw Magic by Kate Magic
Evie's Kitchen by Shazzie

Suppliers and Providers:
www.edenicstates.com

Study Courses:
The College of Living Nutrition.
www.college-living-nutrition.co.uk
Study to become a qualified Living Nutrition Practitioner. The course includes material closely related to the subject matter of this book. Holly is an occasional lecturer on this course.

Education:
www.thetruthaboutcancer.com
www.mercola.com

Raw Supplies:
www.funkyraw.com

Restorative shamanic retreats in nature:
www.livingcleanibogaine.com

Melatonin:
pureencapsulations.com
biovea.co.uk
organicpharmacy.org
asphalia.co.uk: for a natural version or small doses,, this product is made from natural grasses which happen to be rich in melatonin.

Montmorency Cherries
www.cherryactive.co.uk

Wellsprings Serenity cream.
http://www.wellsprings-serenity.com/

Raw Dairy Suppliers

Case for untreated milk:
www.seedsofhealth.co.uk/articles/case_for_untreated_milk.shtml

About the heat treatment of milk:
Thermised milk is raw milk that has been heated for at least 15 seconds at a temperature between 57 °C and 68 °C. Pasteurisation is a process by which milk is is heated to 71.7 °C for 15–20 seconds. So pasteurisation involves higher temperatures than thermisation but both processes heat the milk to above biological temperature and damage important nutrients and biological factors. Many cheeses described as 'unpasteurised' are in fact thermised and therefore not truly raw; it's worth checking with the supplier if you want genuinely raw cheese.

In the UK:

www.hookandson.co.uk raw organic cows milk and butter delivered to your door anywhere in the country
Emma's Organic Dairy – organic raw milk in the north of England and throughout the UK; Rare Breed Shorthorn Cows, superior quality natural milk
Beaconhill Farm fresh unpasteurised jersey cows milk and cream, mail order around the country. To order, call 01531 640 275 or 07986 329 081. John farms in an organic manner i.e. no artificial fertilizer, no pesticides and no prophylactic antibiotics (Dry Cow Therapy).
Dreamers Farm deliveries of raw Jersey cows milk in Glastonbury area. Jersey milk is exceptionally nutritious.
Milky Business are a supplier of raw milk in Nottinghamshire, East Midlands. Plainspot Farm, Plainspot Road, Brinsley, Nottingham, NG16 5BQ 07970839991
Hurdlebrook Farm Raw milk and cheese from Guernsey cows in Babcary, Somerset and online.

Blackburne & Haynes Meadow Cottage, Churt Rd, Headley, Bordon 01428 712155 Raw jersey agrochemical-free milk.
Lubcloud Dairy, raw cows milk from farm or delivered.
Blessed Organic: raw organic milk delivery, all over the country, cold and fresh, within hours of milking. http://organicrawmilk.co.uk/raw-organic-milk-delivery/ delivery in London on Monday ring Max 07877315216
Wheelbirks Dairy Farm High and Tom Richardson, Stockseld, Northumberland NE43 7HY, 0661 842613, 07717 282014 buy milk at the farm or contact them for delivery, Jersey cows
Modbury Farm, Dorset, delicious raw jersey milk available from the farm shop.
Plaw Hatch Farm, Forest Row, biodynamic raw milk and cream from cows with horns!
Plawhatch Lane, Sharpthorne, East Grinstead, West Sussex RH19 4JL, 01342 810652
Raw sheep milk, Top Paddock Dairy, Horsham, Sussex,www.sheepdairy.co.uk
Raw goats milk: Bevital Biodynamic goats milk sent out frozen by mail order. www.bevital.co.uk
Raw milk: Slack House Farm, Gilsland, Cumbria, tel 016977 47351 www.slackhousefarm.co.uk
Raw Goats' Cheese: truckles of Allerdale available mail order from Thornby Moor Dairy, Crofton Hall, Thursby, Carslisle, CA5 6QB, Cumbria, 01697 345555

Raw cheese (not all of their cheeses are raw) at Country Cheeses, shops in Totnes, Tavistock and Topsham or shipped out, you can email or phone them: www.countrycheeses.co.uk
Raw (unpasteurised) goats, ewe's and cows cheese in Better Foods shop, Bristol.
Raw Cheese at Ben's Farm Shop, Staverton, Devon.
Raw milk, cheese and butter at red23
www.red23.co.uk/Raw-Unpasteurised-Dairy_c_60.html

Yoghurt made from raw milk cannot legally be sold in shops although you can make it yourself at home very easily by mixing a couple of spoonfuls live yoghurt with body warm milk and leaving in a thermos ask overnight. Kefir is easier to make and is a more powerful form of yoghurt so can be used as well. Kefir cultures are available at various outlets online.
Cheese Starter: available from Moorlands Cheesemakers: www.cheesemaking.co.uk
Other Raw Dairy Producers listed www.seedsofhealth.co.uk/resources/dairy/index.shtml
and www.meetup.com/westonaprice-london/about
www.meetup.com/westonaprice-london/pages/Mail_Order/ also www.naturalfoodnder.co.uk/unpasteurised-raw-milk-uk
for more info on obtaining raw milk in the UK visit www.realmilk.com/where- other.html#uk
In France:
This website has a map of all the raw milk dispensers throughout France: www.distrilait.fr/implantations-producteurs-concessionnaires-distrilait/
In the US:
go to www.rawmilk.org/
For information on obtaining raw milk worldwide:
visit www.realmilk.com.
Cheeses that are generally raw (check the label) include gruyère, emmental, brie de meaux, and roquefort.

Appendix 1

B17 in foods

Keep in mind that these are averages only and that specimens vary widely depending on variety, locale, soil, and climate.

Fruits and their range
blackberry, domestic low
blackberry, wild high
boysenberry med.
choke cherry high
wild crabapple high
market cranberry low
Swedish (lignon) cranberry high
currant med.
elderberry med. to high
gooseberry med.
huckleberry med.
loganberry med.
mulberry med.
quince med.
raspberry med.

Seeds and their range
apple seeds high
apricot seed high
buckwheat med.
cherry seed high
flax med.
millet med.
nectarine seed high

peach seed high
pear seeds high
plum seed high
prune seed high
squash seeds med.

Beans and their range
black low
black-eyed peas low
fava high
garbanzo low to med.
green pea low
kidney low to med.
lentils med.
lima, U.S. low
lima, Burma med.
mung med. to high
shell low
Nuts (all raw) Range*
bitter almond high
cashew low
macadamia med. to high

Sprouts and their range
alfalfa med.
bamboo high
fava med.
garbanzo med.
mung med.
Leaves Range*
alfalfa high
beet tops low
eucalyptus high

spinach low
water cress low

Tubers and their range
cassava high
sweet potato low
yams low

Much of this material on B17 is taken from a paper by Ernst Theodor Krebs, Jr. which was presented in German before a congress of the International Medical Society for Blood and Tumor Disease,
Baden, West Germany. On this occasion, the author received an award honouring his discovery and research on vitamin B-15 (pangamic acid) and vitamin B-17 (nitriloside).

Appendix 2

Foods to Avoid with MAO Inhibitors

(A few hours before and afterwards)

Mono-amine Oxidase Inhibitors stop Monoamine oxidase enzymes working. A side-effect of this is that the amino acid tyramine is also not broken down properly and this can cause unpleasant symptoms and even be dangerous. By taking care, these problems can easily be avoided.

The following categories of food may contain substantial amounts of tyramine and should be avoided:

Alcohol
Banana Peel
Bean Curd (Tofu)
Beans and Peas
Brazils
Cheese
Coconuts
Fish
Ginseng
Miso
Peanuts
Protein Extracts
Meat
Sauerkraut
Shrimp Paste
Soups if they contain miso or protein extracts
Soy Sauce
Tofu
Tempeh

Yeasts
Spoiled, old or fermented food

Foods to be Consumed in only Small Quantities:

Aubergines
Avocados
Caffeine
Chocolate
Figs
Other Dairy Products
Nuts
Pineapple
Raspberries
Red Plums
Soy Sauce
Spinach

Appendix 3

Left and Right Hemispheres the Evidence

Hormonal Retardation and the fall from grace

There are currently some fascinating and ground-breaking results coming of Cambridge University. Professor Simon Baron-Cohen has researching the effects of hormones on brain growth and behaviour. He is best known for his work on autism, including his theory that autism is an extreme form of the "male brain". He has added to the growing body of evidence that testosterone retards the neural development of the left side of the brain and this detrimentally alters behaviour. Interestingly it is his cousin, Sasha Baron-Cohen who creates for the screen such extreme examples of the retarded human behaviour in question. A talented family.

The so-called 'masculisation' of the brain is effectively damage to the left hemisphere of the brain. It is the steroid hormone estradiol that causes this. Estradiol is made from testosterone by the enzyme aromatase. The degree of masculisation therefore is affected by the amount of free testosterone available and the degree of aromatase activity. This damage has occurred to all our left hemispheres – it is just more pronounced in general in men and also some individuals due to higher levels of testosterone. These two factors could account for the higher frequency of left-handedness, also the greater range of intelligence levels including both genius and learning disabilities in males.

The activity of aromatase is inhibited by plant flavonoids and also melatonin. Humans are currently experiencing a deficit of both flavonoids and melatonin. This leads to more aromatase activity, which in turn leads to increased masculisation of the brain and, at the extreme end of the spectrum, autism which is on the increase. (Autism is of course a complex syndrome with probably many factors involved but it seems this is a major one.)

Flavonoids

The research of Katherine Milton on the dietary ecology of primates, human ancestors and modern humans shows how much lower in important plant compounds our diet is now compared with ancestral diets and those of other primates. Studies by her on primate nutrition suggest we have lost more than 95% of the complex plant chemicals and nutrients that fuelled our development as human beings. We know that in the past our diet would have included abundant amount of fruit and that the flavonoids in fruit inhibit the activity of aromatase. The likely link between a change in diet over the millennia and the retardation of the left hemisphere of the brain can be clearly seen.

Flavonoids are known as endocrine disrupters – as we have seen they change the hormonal balance in our brains and bodies. And this changes the way DNA is read to build a baby in it's mother's womb. There are many examples of how a change in hormone levels can affect transcription of DNA and change our bodies and brains. The transformation at puberty is an obvious one. There is an illustration of the power of a change in the way the DNA is read at www.beyond-belief.org.uk.

There are parallels with the transformation of a worker bee into a queen by the increased ingestion of royal jelly. The epigenetic effect of royal jelly on a worker bee during the development of a single generation is quite astounding. If a chemical cocktail with the ability to effectively re-interpret the way the DNA code is read were present 24/7 during the evolution of an organism the results would be equally spectacular. A complete re-design and re-engineering at a molecular and cellular level through to a major re-organisation of development, form and function.

Melatonin

Our original higher flavonoid levels kept our neurotransmitter levels higher because many of them are monoamine oxidase inhibitors. These stimulated the pineal gland to produce more of its hormones including melatonin. Currently the pineal is chronically under-active and are melatonin levels are lower than would be optimal for our day to day health and the transcribing (reading) of the DNA blueprint. This is one reason melatonin is anti-ageing.

References:

Elevated rates of testosterone-related disorders in women with autism spectrum conditions
Erin Ingudomnukul, Simon Baron-Cohen, Sally Wheelwright, Rebecca Knickmeyer

The Empathy Quotient: An Investigation of Adults with Asperger Syndrome or High Functioning Autism, and Normal Sex Differences
Simon Baron-Cohen and Sally Wheelwright

Terence McKenna on iboga:
www.youtube.com/watch?v=-uM2At8JbSI

Cerebral dominance: the biological foundations
by Norman Geschwind and Albert M. Galaburda 1984

Papers by Katherine Milton:

Back to Basics: Why Foods of Wild Primates have Relevance for Modern Human Health
Katherine Milton PhD

Nutritional Characteristics of Wild Primate foods: Do the Diets of our Closest Living Relatives Have Lessons for Us
Micronutrient intakes of wild primates: are humans different?
Katherine Milton

A stroke of insight

www.youtube.com/watch?v=UyyjU8fzEYU
www.ted.com/talks/view/id/229

Neuroanatomist Jill Bolte Taylor had an opportunity few brain scientists would wish for: One morning, she realized she was having a massive stroke. As it happened — as she felt her brain functions slip away one by one, speech, movement, understanding — she studied and remembered every moment. This is a powerful story about how our brains define us and connect us to the world and to one another.

Note that the stroke was to the left hemisphere. Her experiences therefore give many clues as to the roles of the hemispheres. However we do need to be aware that the right hemisphere is not running at its full potential in any of us, due to a lifetime of suppression by the left hemisphere and also not receiving the total nutrition and fuel it requires to run on. When left hemisphere function is lost, we get a glimpse into the potential of the right hemisphere but we do not see its full potential straight away. So having to manage with a damaged left hemisphere caused Jill Bolte Taylor problems initially. As Jill Bolte Taylor found, in the years after her stroke she recovered lost function and gained abilities she had not had before.

'In response to the swelling and trauma of the stroke, which placed pressure on her dominant left hemisphere, the functions of her right hemisphere blossomed'.

She is now known as the 'The Singing Scientist'.

Her website is here: drjilltaylor.com.

Jill Bolte Taylor's experiences hint at the kind of latent potential of our brains - and show what is potentially available when the left hemisphere's stranglehold is removed.

Extraordinary Talents
Autistic Savants and other Extraordinary People

Autistic savants comprise a very small percentage of the autistic population but their enhanced capabilities along with those of some people whose left hemisphere has been damaged show what potential function there is when the constraints of the left hemisphere are even partially lifted.

From Left in the Dark by Tony Wright:

"...one nine year-old boy was transformed from an 'ordinary' school child to a genius mechanic after a bullet destroyed a part of his left hemisphere. Ten year-old Orlando Serrell also acquired uncanny abilities after a baseball struck him on the left side of the head. After the injury healed, he found he could perform calendar calculations of baffling complexity and also recall the weather, where he was and what he was doing for every day since the accident. His feats made the news headlines."

In yet more cases, five patients from the Californian School of Medicine developed amazing drawing skills after dementia destroyed some specific parts of the left side of their brains. One of them had spent his life fitting car stereos and had never shown an interest in art. When dementia destroyed neurones in his left front temporal cortex, he suddenly started to produce sensational images depicting scenes from his early childhood. It was as if the destruction of those brain cells took the brakes off some innate ability that had been suppressed for most of his life.

These unlocked abilities parallel the astounding numerical, musical and artistic skills of autistic savants, memorably portrayed by Dustin Hoffman in the film 'Rain Man'. There is a well-documented real life case in which this sort of heightened ability has reached a quite phenomenal level. Stephen Wiltshire is an autistic savant. He has severe learning difficulties yet, despite huge deficits, he has an extraordinary talent for drawing. At the age of eleven, he drew the Natural History Museum and other notable London landmarks to such a high standard that the well-known architect/artist Sir Hugh Casson described him as "the best child artist in Britain".

But it is Stephen's memory that is so astounding. At the age of 15, for a television documentary, he was taken for a half-hour helicopter ride over London. He took no notes or photographs and yet, back on the ground, he was able to produce a totally accurate aerial drawing of four square miles of the capital, incorporating over 200 buildings. His pencil never stopped, and he never corrected his work. It could be argued that London was already familiar to him; but he recently performed exactly the same feat in Rome, this time reproducing an accurate panorama of the entire city on a wall-mounted six metre long roll of paper.

Stephen Wiltshire's combination of photographic memory and highly accomplished draughtsmanship is an extraordinary, almost preternatural faculty. And yet it may be simply an extreme manifestation of a skill-set we all possess. It is possible that somewhere within all our brains there is the ability to mentally 'photograph' all the detail that we see. We normally filter out this detail, as it is either not relevant or too complicated for the dominant part of the brain to cope with.

Most experts assume that this left brain filtration system is necessary to enable us to focus on our thinking. The left brain just cannot cope with the mass of detail so, in order to function at all, it either has to filter most of it out or not process it in the first place. So where is a photographic memory like Stephen Wiltshire's stored? Almost certainly in the right hemisphere or at least facilitated by its operation. ...

There is some evidence that suggests that the right hemisphere may be even better with language than the left. The autistic savant Daniel Tammet can not only perform extraordinary mathematical calculations at breakneck speeds but, unlike other savants who can perform similar feats, he speaks seven languages (French, German, Spanish, Lithuanian, Icelandic and Esperanto) and is even devising his own – "Mänti". Icelandic is a very difficult language to learn and yet Daniel Tammet mastered it within a week. Though there are many theories about savants, it is usual that some kind of brain damage causes the affliction – perhaps the onset of dementia later in life, a blow to the head or, in the case of Daniel, an epileptic fit when he was three.

Scans of the brains of autistic savants suggest that the right hemisphere might be compensating for damage in the left hemisphere. There is therefore the possibility that, in Daniel's case, his right hemisphere is giving him his outstanding language ability (as well as the ability to calculate cube roots quicker than an electronic calculator and recall Pi to 22,514 decimal places). If it is indeed right hemisphere processing that is giving Tammet his facility with language then, even if the right has compensated for a breakdown of the left, it somehow processes languages better than a normal left hemisphere can. Does this mean that the right has magically grown ultra proficient or are its skills inherent and normally kept bottled up by left hemisphere dominance? ...

Other unusual things happen to our language skills too when the dominant hemisphere is left without the support of the right. For instance, in Sturge-Weber syndrome when the right hemisphere is irreparably damaged, speech is typically delivered in a monotone and even the difference between male and female voices becomes impossible to discern.

In one bizarre case, a nine year-old boy suddenly learnt how to speak after his left hemisphere was removed. 'Alex' was born with a disorder called Sturge-Weber syndrome, which disrupted the blood supply to the left side of his brain. He suffered epileptic fits and could only utter a few indistinct sounds; his only intelligible word was 'mama'. He was so ill that doctors decided that the only way his fits could be controlled was by removing the damaged half of the brain. Most remarkably, two years after the surgery Alex could talk like a normal child. This result caused quite a stir because, according to accepted theory, we can only acquire language during the first few years of our lives. Most people who start to speak unusually late never become very proficient. As we grow older it seems that our brains lose 'plasticity' – networks of nerve cells lose the ability to form new connections on which learning depends.

Darold Treffert, Clinical Professor at University of Wisconsin Medical School, has studied savant syndrome for over forty years. His book 'Extraordinary People' was the first comprehensive summary of autistic savant syndrome and is probably the world authority on autistic savants. In a recent statement he has said: 'I've come more and more to the conclusion that rather than there being right hemisphere compensation, there is rather release from the 'tyranny' of the left hemisphere'

Links:

The Boy With The Incredible Brain
http://video.google.com/videoplay?docid=4913196365903075662#

Beautiful Mind: Stephen Wiltshire (autistic savant)
http://www.youtube.com/watch?v=dAfaM_CBvP8

The Rainman Twins
http://www.youtube.com/watch?v=f5IAecvEA-4

Savant Syndrome: An extraordinary Condition Darold A Treffert MD
www.wisconsinmedicalsociety.org/system/files/savant_article.pdf

Darold Treffert
http://www.daroldtreffert.com/

Enhanced Brain Function
Allan Snyder's work on enhanced brain function

In the 1990's Professor Allan Snyder at the Centre of the Mind in Australia began conducting research involving temporarily shutting down the left temporal lobe of the brain using transcranial magnetic stimulation. During the experiments enhanced artistic and mathematical ability and improved memory emerge.

The skills that emerged in Allan Snyder's experiments mirror those of autistic savants and also occur in some people whose left hemisphere has been damaged.

In Snyder's words: "You could call this a creativity-amplifying machine. It's a way of altering our states of mind without taking drugs like mescaline. You can make people see the raw data of the world as it is. As it is actually represented in the unconscious mind of all of us." A number of Allan Snyder's subjects have reported perceptual changes too – feelings of euphoria and bliss more normally associated with 'peak experiences' and meditation.

Links:

Savant-like numerosity skills revealed in normal people by magnetic pulses: Allan Snyder, Homayoun Bahramali, Tobias Hawker, D John, May 2006 Mitchell

http://www.perceptionweb.com/abstract.cgi?id=p5539

Savant for a Day   Lawrence Osborne
New your times Magazine   June 22 2003

http://www.wireheading.com/brainstim/savant.html

A Sensed Presence

Michael Persinger - Psychotropic drugs and nature of reality

This is a fascinating lecture by Michael Persinger:
video.google.com/videoplay?docid=4292093832329014323

Michael Persinger has been a professor at Laurentian University, Ontario, Canada since 1971 and has written numerous papers and six books including 'The Neuropsychological Base of God Beliefs'. One of his most significant areas of research has been on the effects of magnetic fields on perception.

In 1987, he began systematically testing trial subjects with complex electro-magnetic fields after discovering that they could induce a number of experiences, ranging from a sensed presence to religious and mystical feelings. His aims were to determine which portions of the brain, or its electro-magnetic patterns, generate the experiences. The results of the experiments clearly show differences between the left and right hemispheres. Euphoric, religious or mystical experiences were accessed when the right hemisphere was stimulated. Furthermore, the sense of something or someone present seemed to be a left hemisphere interpretation of the intrusion from the right hemisphere. This 'sensed presence' was often interpreted (by the subject's left hemisphere) as spirits, ghosts, angels, gods, devils or aliens. Again it seems that the left hemisphere is trying its (limited) best here to attach some concept, however unlikely, to a numinous right hemisphere experience.

Particularly of interest is the way psychedelic drugs imitate the effects of certain neurotransmitters to affect the brain, for example LSD imitates serotonin and mescaline imitates dopamine. It is not the substance itself that is experienced but the boosting of the brain's own neurochemistry. Persinger mimicked the effects of these kinds of substances with weak electromagnetic fields. The temporal pattern of the fields corresponded to the molecular structures of the compounds. Interestingly psychedelic substances do not produce altered states of consciousness in people who have lost the use of the right hemisphere, just as the electromagnetic fields have a particular effect on the right hemisphere. And as with psychedelic drugs it takes 15-20 minutes for the electromagnetic fields to produce an effect.

This article is a very interesting description of an encounter with Michael Persinger's research:

This Is Your Brain on God by Jack Hitt
'Michael Persinger has a vision – the Almighty isn't dead, he's an energy field. And your mind is an electromagnetic map to your soul'.

http://www.wired.com/wired/archive/7.11/persinger.html

Tall Tales

Anosognosia is a condition in which a person who suffers disability seems unaware of or denies the existence of his or her disability (wikipedia). It can occur after brain injury or other neurological impairment. Anosognosia occurs in over half of right hemisphere stroke patients (J. Cutting put the figure at 58% in a study described in 1978), while it hardly ever occurs in left hemisphere stroke victims.

The right hemisphere of our brain is the part which directly perceives the complexity of reality. The left brain relies on conceptualisations which can only ever be an approximation to reality. The left brain relies on new information updates from the right brain to refresh its views on what is happening. Without this input it stays stuck in the same beliefs and story lines which become increasingly divorced from on-going reality.

Confabulation is the formation of false memories, perceptions, or beliefs... as a result of neurological dysfunction (wikipedia). It leads to a situation where people lie without realising they are lying. Clearly this can happen as a result of anosognosia.

Modern humans are all dominated by the left brain, particularly in terms of thought and speech, and the right hemisphere has to take a back seat, its impressions becoming sub-conscious. Therefore we do not consciously perceive full reality. And, as part of this very scenario, we are not habitually aware of this limitation. We could all be said to be suffering from partial anosognosia. This is why we all confabulate to some degree. This was highlighted in an article in New Scientist in October 2006 (available at http://www.newscientist.com/.

The Evolutionary Biology of Self-Deception,
Laughter, Dreaming and Depression: Some Clues from Anosognosia
http://leftinthedark.org.uk/PDF/Ramachandran%20VS%20Evol.pdf

Appendix 4

Tenets of Redemptive Religion

There are four main facets to redemptive religion:

Belief in an off-planet paternalistic creator, a father God, who creates humanity without a consort and oversees it.

Belief in a chosen people - a group of people chosen to represent the paternalistic god and fulfil his destiny.

Belief in a messiah sent by the paternalistic god to save the people because they can't live up to his insane rules.

Belief in a day of judgement, a doomsday, an apocalypse, when judgement is pronounced because humanity still can't get it right.

We can apply this principle to many groups who feel they have got it right (are righteous).
There is a difference between authentically feeling right in the sense of feeling good in yourself and having the belief that you are right above others (righteousness).
Righteousness is linked to the quest for perfection, a theoretical point of infinitesimally small magnitude which we can never reach and has nothing to do with life.